Diary of a Sex Doctor

The sexual experiences of my patients and the consequences of those experiences

Michael D. McKane M.D.

A&B Publishers Group
Brooklyn, New York
11238

Diary of a Sex Doctor

Michael D. McKane M.D.

A&B Publishers Group
Brooklyn, New York
11238

Published by
A&B PUBLISHERS GROUP
Upstream publications division
1000 Atlantic Avenue.
Brooklyn, NY 11238.

Distributed by
📖 A&B DISTRIBUTORS INC.,
1000 Atlantic Avenue.
Brooklyn, NY 11238.

Diary of A Sex Doctor © 2003 By Michael D. McKane. Printed and bound in Canada. All rights reserved. No part of this book may be reproduced or transmitted in any form or by any means including electronic, mechanical or photocopying or recording or stored in a retrieval system without permission in writing from the publisher except by a reviewer who may quote brief passage to be included in a review.

ISBN: 1-881316-27-0

The contents of this book are for the purposes of education and information.

COVER DESIGN: *A & B PUBLISHERS GROUP*

04 05 06 07..08 09 10   9 8 7 6 5 4 3 2 1
Printed in Canada

CONTENTS

Introduction – vii
1. It can happen to *You!* 1
2. It Can Happen to Anyone Around You! 10
3. God's Scourge? 19
4. Symptoms? 26
5. Protect Yourself! But How? 30
6. More Patients 30
7. Some Facts and Fallacies About STD's 45
8. A Reflection 50
9. More Cases 52
10. Syphilis 65
11. Venereal Warts 73
12. When Sex is Deadly 84
13. A Doctor's Role in the Treatment of STDs 91

14. When Sex is *Not* Life-Affirming 97
15. When a Harmless Fetish Can Be Dangerous.................108
16. When Love Hurts, and That's How He Likes It 119
17. Sometimes It's Just a Matter of Trust.............................129
18. When Sex Equals Disease...135
19. In Search of a Fantasy Fulfilled 141
20. Teachers and Students..153
21. That Locker Room Syndrome 162
22. When There's No Sex at Home 167
23. When Sex *Shouldn't* Happen — and the Consequences183
Conclusion — 149

Introduction

The alarm rang, as it does every morning, at precisely 5:17 a.m. Before I opened my eyes, my arm reached out from beneath the blanket and moved in a practiced fashion to the clock where my fingers found the button on the alarm. Although I was still half-asleep, there was no restless groping at the clock. If nothing else, my rigorous training through internship and residency had prepared me to be remarkably exact under the most trying of circumstances. Still, a shotgun wound at three in the morning is sometimes easier to deal with than the damn alarm...

"What time is it?" my wife asked sleepily.

"Go back to sleep," I said softly as I started to slide out from under the blanket.

"Uh-huh," she sighed, turning over and closing her eyes again as my feet touched the cold floor.

I put on my robe and slippers and went into the kitchen. I filled the coffee maker with water and then headed into the bathroom. The bright light in the bathroom took a moment to adjust to. Once my eyes were comfortable with the light, I stood in front of the sink and observed my reflection in the mirror. Resting my hands on the cool, white porcelain I studied my face. Not as young as I was but not old either. Hmm. Not bad. A few lines. They give me a weathered, serious look. The gray in my hair? A certain touch of years and wisdom.

I wondered what my patients thought when they looked at me. Did they see someone who cared about them? Who wanted to help them? Or did they see just a generic face, one that represented the medical establishment to them?

The interesting thing is, I have genuine sympathy and caring for my patients. I can't remember a single patient who I didn't *feel* something for, for whom I didn't have some respect for their struggles.

And my patients *do* struggle. They don't come to me like they come to other physicians. A person calls her doctor and says she has a fever. Her doctor treats her. There is never any fear of judgment. But my patients come to me not only with physical ailments and diseases but too often with a sense of shame at how they acquired their diseases. I understand their emotions. My task is to aid them not only heal their bodies but to ease their minds as well. I often must assure them that their illness is not some cruel "divine retribution" for some sinful behavior or some other such nonsense... but it is not nonsense if my patients struggle against it.

And that's much of the point. My patients come to me with what is politely termed, in other contexts "baggage".

I try to do everything I can to ease their suffering — of both body and soul.

I turned on the hot water and lathered my hands with soap. I take great care when I wash my hands. Washing hands is an occupational necessity. It is also a habit that carries over into my personal life.

After showering and shaving, I returned to the kitchen for

coffee and a light breakfast. By six I have eaten, read the paper, dressed and, in my mind, reviewed the patients I had seen the day before.

I was ready to begin another day.

I left the house and stepped out onto the porch. I paused for a moment to breathe in the fresh, morning air. As I did, I looked up and down the block.

I live on a street of comfortable, well-tended houses. The gardens are neat. The lawns mowed. Most of the houses have at least two cars in their driveway. It is a normal, clean, nice neighborhood. Many of my neighbors are professionals. Lawyers. Accountants. A publisher. Two psychologists. Another doctor. We greet each other and exchange pleasantries. They all know that I am a dermatologist.

What they don't know is that my practice is not the same as most dermatologists. I do not see patients with acne or everyday rashes. In my practice I treat patients who, because of the maladies they suffer from, choose to come to a hospital clinic rather than their private physicians. I treat patients who suffer from sexually transmitted diseases (STD's). The reality of sexuality and sexual practice in America today makes me more than the one who treats their physical conditions. In my practice, I am often called upon to be physician, counselor, advisor and confessor.

In a society nearly crippled with ambivalent mores and hypocrisies, I must be a true healer.

I am, in actuality, a sex doctor.

In my nice neighborhood my neighbors might be shocked by the realities of my practice. A sex doctor on their block? They might shudder at their perception of the patients I might see during my hospital rounds, the men and women who suffer from sexually transmitted diseases, diseases often gotten during furtive and illicit sexual adventures.

Who might they imagine I treat? Prostitutes and others of "immoral character"? The poor? The homeless? No doubt they presume my patients are people of color or of immigrant backgrounds.

They would not be wrong. However, they would be profoundly wrong to believe that those are my only patients. They would be wrong to presume that my patients do not live in this neighborhood and in hundreds... thousands more just like it.

Many of my neighbors might believe the beauty of the facade our nice, neat neighborhood presents. They might take solace in the belief that membership in a country club or sending children to the "right" school can hold sexually transmitted diseases at bay. They might have faith that the diseases that my patients suffer with do not live here, among the rolling lawns and colorful flower beds. My neighbors would be wrong to do so.

If they believe that the sexual urges that ultimately bring people to me are held at bay by rolling lawns and white picket fences they would be profoundly mistaken.

The patients I see and the diseases they struggle with live here. Indeed, they are right at home here. Just as they are in *barrios* and ghettos, in urban centers and rural farms.

New York City might be well-known as a modern "Sodom and Gomorra" but the same sexual expression that is prominent in New York exists in Minnesota and Iowa, in Kansas and South Dakota.

I have learned from medical experience that the basic urges that my patients respond to are not limited by geography, socio-economic demographics, ethnic background or gender. Sex and sexuality is a primal drive that defines much of our lives—either in how we embrace it or how we deny it. Most often we are defined by the balance we are forced to make between the two extremes of that spectrum.

Certainly the patients you will hear from in these pages have. I will allow their stories and their voices to speak with you. I believe that they, and not I, can put a human face on the struggle for sexual expression, sexual experience and, too often, sexually transmitted diseases.

Ultimately, that is what this book is about—sexually transmitted diseases. While many sexual adventures cause emotional turmoil and have social repercussions (especially when they are of an extramarital nature), it is the physical havoc that they have the potential to cause that we need to look at.

For this, the STD's, are preventable.

As you will hear in the voices of my patients, their sexual experiences come from deep needs, needs we all share. However, they end up with me because their sexual adventures resulted in disease.

As I have said, none of us should consider "casting the first stone" of judgment against these people. They are like us. They *are* us. None of us is immune to desire and none of us is protected from acted on that desire if we find ourselves in circumstances that are new to us.

And, ultimately, as we will discover, it is often the neglect of our "monogamous" sexual partners that creates the real possibility for sexual adventurism outside the bounds of that relationship.

Listen to their voices. Do not be offended by their words or their blunt descriptions. Listen to the drive that animates their experiences.

You will hear your voice.

1

It can happen to *You!*

Sarah (not her real name) sat across my desk from me and nervously toyed with her pearl necklace. Her manner and her dress indicated that she was a successful businesswoman, which I later found out was the case. In fact, she had started her own small advertising business only a few years earlier.

"It was a lot of work," she confessed to me during our initial conversation. "My relationship with my husband suffered—not that things were going so well before the business. The kids were more understanding, frankly. Both my daughters were proud of me for finally *doing something* with my life. Robert didn't understand though. I think he felt threatened on some level. After all, he felt that he made a good enough living. Why should I have to work? Even when I explained that with the girls both in college I was ready for something more in my life than simply being a housewife he didn't understand.

"He tried to be humorous about it in the beginning. He began to introduce me to at parties as his *working* wife. As if my working was a novelty."

"It sounds like a very difficult time in your relationship," I observed.

She sighed. "Yes. Yes, it was difficult. But the reality was that even when our relationship wasn't quite so difficult it was hardly good." She shrugged. "We hadn't been particularly intimate for a long while. Once I began working..." She let the thought trail off.

"The separation was relatively amicable," she added with a quick, almost embarrassed smile. "Actually, we made a much better separated couple than we did a married couple. Ironic, isn't it?"

I returned her smile. It was ironic. And sad. Unfortunately, it wasn't that unusual. Too many couples finally get along better when their presumptions about one another are altered and they are forced to be honest.

"After the separation, I totally devoted myself to work. There were days when I never even came up for air. It was quite a roller coaster ride. Just when my life seemed to be falling apart on a personal level, professionally things were really taking off.

"Still, after a few months, my friends insisted that I stop being so focused on work. They suggested that I begin to date. They said I had become more boring than when I was just a housewife." She shrugged. "That hit me where it hurt. So I went on a couple of dates friends set up for me." Sarah glanced down at her hands in her lap. "They were so awkward. I mean, I hadn't been on a date in more than twenty years. Dinner and the movies—fine. I have always had a number of male friends and we get along fine. But kissing? Making out? Come on, that was for my daughters, not for me." She laughed and threw back her shoulder-length brown hair which was just beginning to show gray highlights. "My God, I was forty-seven!"

I liked Sarah. She spoke with refreshing candor.

She shrugged again. "Still, there was something exciting about being *out there* again. I hadn't thought of myself as attractive for a long time—certainly not in that way. I guess that was one of the results of my marriage and being taken for granted. So it felt *good* to have men looking at me, at my body. A little unnerving at times, true, but in a good way.

"I started working out at the gym. Over the next few months, it was flattering to find out how many men were interested in spending time with me. But the idea of actually having sex with anyone... I just couldn't imagine it. The practicalities completely unhinged me. Looking good in clothes was one thing. But being alone with someone again. Undoing my bra or worse, having someone else undo it. Being naked in front of someone other than Robert...

"And I didn't even know how to think of having a man naked with me. After all those years of marriage, I felt as unskilled and naive as a virgin.

"And, truth be known, even with my visits to the gym and the fact that I always tried to keep in reasonably good shape but there's no question that the years take their toll....

"I guess the dating was having some effect though. In spite of my doubts and worries, I was thinking of romance and sex more than I had in years. I might not have quite figured out how to deal with being naked with a man again but I was definitely thinking about it.

"One weekend, I attended a magnificent wedding reception. It was gorgeous. The bride's parents did everything with such elegance. The guests all seemed as elegant as the setting. One gentleman, Michael, introduced himself to me toward the end of the evening and asked me to dance.

"He was utterly charming. Like me, he was recently separated. He was honest with his ambivalence about what had happened. Took some of the blame. Confessed how uncomfortable he was being out `on the hunt' again. He used those very words, `out on the hunt'. He laughed easily. He said he felt awkward at weddings, knowing what he did about marriage. I laughed with him.

"`The things I could tell the bride...' I joked. `I'll bet,' he replied.

"Before leaving, he asked for my phone number and I gave it to him without any hesitation. I didn't think he'd call though. Maybe I just wanted him to. But he did call, the next day. We went out the following weekend. Dinner in a nice restaurant. Coffee. We talked for a long time and then he took me home. He seemed not to expect anything so there was no awkwardness. I appreciated that.

"We dated casually for a couple of months with little more than a peck on the cheek and a friendly hug. And then he asked if I wanted to go to the Cape with him for a weekend. I was taken by surprise. I mean, we'd become more friendly—holding hands and touching each other casually when we laughed—but we'd hardly been intimate. But I thought, *Why not?* We were both adults after all."

Sarah colored slightly. "The weekend was marvelous. I hadn't felt like that in a long, long time. He enjoyed things my husband never did, like performing oral sex on me. I.. I was happy to reciprocate." She colored a bit deeper and smiled in embarrassment.

"And so here I am," she said, lowering her eyes.

"*That's* why you're here?" I asked her. "You're here because you had oral sex and you enjoyed it?"

"Not exactly. Not that alone," she conceded.

"Tell me exactly why you're here," I prompted her gently.

"A week to ten days after we were at the Cape, I developed cold sores in my mouth. I'd had cold sores before so at first I didn't give them much thought. But then I also began to experience vaginal itching and discharge." She shook her head. "It took me a few very uncomfortable days to put two and two together." She lowered her head. "I can't believe this has happened to me."

I looked at her sympathetically. "Well, I'd like to perform a physical exam and then some lab tests so we can determine exactly what is going on. However, if you are correct in your suspicions I can tell you one thing—what happened to you *can* happen to anyone.

"And it does."

I rang to one of my nurses. "Mary, could you come in my office please?"

Mary is a wonderful nurse, about sixty-two. She looks a bit older. Like a lovely old grandmother. Which is exactly what she is.

Mary escorted Sarah to an examination room. As they left my office, I could hear Mary telling Sarah not to worry, that I was a wonderful doctor and she was sure everything would be all right. I smiled to myself. With nurses like Mary it was hard not to enjoy taking care of patients.

While Sarah was on her way to the examination room, I reviewed the brief notes I had made. Based on what she had told me, I didn't doubt that the examination would show a sexually transmitted disease. However, one of the things that every doctor has to guard against is a sense of complacency in diagnosis. A particular symptom can be the result of a number of conditions.

When I came in a moment later, she was already wearing an examination robe and was on the examination table. "I always said I could wear anything off the rack," she joked, gesturing toward the paper robe. "But I don't know that this is a particularly flattering fit."

I laughed at her joke as I stepped to the metal sink and washed my hands. She was clearly a wonderful, energetic woman who knew how to find enjoyment in life. I was glad to be able to help her.

"Now, let me explain exactly what I'm going to be doing so that you'll know and understand," I said. I took a sealed, cotton swab and, after tearing open the seal, explained that I needed to swab the sores in her mouth. "I'll send this to the lab," I added as I replaced the swab in the wrapper and marked it for the lab.

"Now, if you'll just rest back and place your feet in the stirrups..."

I sat down on an adjustable stool and gently eased Sarah's knees apart. I took note of the discharge that was visible at the entrance to her vagina. "Okay, take an easy breath and try to relax," I said as I took several additional swabs of her vaginal discharge.

Upon physical examination, I found soreness and inflammation in her vagina and urethra. "Have you been experiencing any discomfort when you urinate?" I asked.

"A burning sensation," she admitted. "But not all the time." She lowered her head back until it was resting on the table. "I was hoping it was just a yeast infection," she sighed. "Guess not, huh?"

Sarah's symptoms and eventual lab report indicated the finding I suspected from our initial conversation in my office—that she had contracted gonorrhea during her sexual relations on the Cape.

Because she was still seeing Michael, she was able to confront him with her diagnosis. "I wasn't angry at him. At least, I tried not to be," she told me when she returned for a follow-up visit. "After all, we are both adults. I was a little hurt though." During that conversation, he admitted that he had gone out with a number of different women during the early part of his separation—before he had met Sarah. He had even engaged the services of a prostitute at one point.

"He was obviously embarrassed by having to tell me these things," she explained. "He said he'd just felt so strange, so awkward being single again. He said he was shocked to discover that the women he went out with *expected* to have sex.

"There were a few weeks when he felt this wonderful sense of freedom, when he could live out his fantasies, but then, as he said, he found himself longing for something more than just lust. He said he was looking for a wonderful, beautiful grown-up." She smiled. "He said that's what he found in me."

Michael also swore to Sarah that he hadn't been with another woman since he began dating her.

"He was so charming," Sarah sighed, remembering their first meetings. As if charm was a protection against sexually transmitted diseases.

The reality is that there are very few methods of protection against sexually transmitted diseases. Unfortunately, charm is not among them. Of the methods that do work, the best and most important is knowledge.

As a doctor, my role is two-fold. I try to treat the conditions my patients present to me. I also try to educate my patients so that they will be able to *prevent* suffering disease and discomfort.

"I just feel so stupid," Sarah had said when she was seated on the examination table. She raised her arms helplessly. "I mean, I'm the kind of person who does research before buying a damned blender for the kitchen. I can't believe I let myself get into this situation. I feel like some fifteen year old girl."

"I should have known better..."

"You shouldn't be so hard on yourself," I counseled her. "If you were guilty of anything it was that you were just being a healthy, feeling woman. From what you've told me, you were long overdue for some real romance and passion in your life. There's nothing wrong with that. Nothing at all."

She shrugged. "Thank you. That's very kind of you to say that."

"It's very true. Although we live in a society and culture which often tries to downplay sexual desire the reality is, healthy people have healthy sexual appetites. That is how it should be.

"Healthy sexual appetites do not necessarily mean that we make ourselves vulnerable to STD's though."

Sarah hung her head. "I just never thought it could happen to me..."

None of my patients enter into a sexual relationship thinking that, at some point in that relationship, they will end up in my examination room. Most of us have an inflated sense of our safety. The simple fact is, *none* of us think of becoming the victim of an STD. But STD's cross all lines of race, color, age and economic standing. What's more, because our sexuality is such an intimate aspect of our lives, people who, from the "outside" would seem least vulnerable are often the most vulnerable.

Sarah is a perfect example. To see her on the street, you would probably not consider her sexually active in a relationship that could result in an STD.

So many of the patients I have treated defy the "image" of someone who might have an STD. Yes, I have treated prostitutes and homosexuals. I have treated individuals whose promiscuity place them at high risk for STD. But I have also treated grandmothers and secretaries, bankers and band leaders.

You wouldn't have suspected Sarah of having an STD. The same was true of a patient I treated only a short time before Sarah came to me.

2

It Can Happen to Anyone Around You!

John presented himself to be exactly what the world perceived him to be—the president of a prominent corporation in New York City. At forty-five years of age, he had reached the pinnacle of financial success. He dressed in fine business suits and custom made shirts. At five feet nine inches and one hundred and sixty pounds, he looked to be the physical archetype of the modern, successful man. He appeared to be "on top of the world."

However, as with most appearances, this one was deceptive. While to the outside world, John was the personification of everything they aspired to—position, family, prominence and wealth—John was a good deal more complex than the person people perceived him to be. In addition to the person his family, friends and colleagues knew, John had a secret life only a small handful of people were familiar with.

"This is me," he declared as he handed me an envelope filled with photographs. I took the envelope and looked through the pictures, each one showing an image of a blonde wearing a tight sweater.

I looked at the photographs closely. Although the "woman" in them wore heavy make-up and had broad, masculine shoulders, she was not unattractive. I handed the photographs back to John. He was watching me closely.

"That's me," he said again, nodding to the photographs. "I'm Linda." I looked at photographs again and then at him. He smiled at me with some degree of self-consciousness. Then I glanced back at a photograph he had taken from the envelope and placed laying face up on the desk. It *was* him.

"I keep these in my personal safe at work," he said, returning the photograph to the manila envelope. "I can't even imagine what happen if the people I know found out about me."

John. Successful businessman. Husband of twenty years. Father of two young children. Transvestite.

"Maria, my wife, doesn't suspect a thing about my secret life," he said, his voice dropping to a conspiratorial whisper. "It's funny though. In a sad way. Of all the people in my life, she would probably be the one who might understand. She'd probably try anyway."

He spoke of his wife with obvious warmth and caring. It was clear to me that they enjoyed a loving relationship. He obviously adored his children, whom he described as "gorgeous and wonderful." When he showed me pictures of them, the younger of the two, a girl, bore a striking resemblance to the "Linda" I had seen in the earlier photographs.

"Curious, isn't it?" he said, commenting upon the way his face looked more like his daughter's when he was in make-up. "It's a strange world," he added somewhat mysteriously. Then he shrugged.

The more we spoke, the more I found him to be a warm, kind and considerate man with a quick sense of humor. He tended toward introspection and displayed the gift for real empathy toward others. Although he had often been harassed as "Linda" he was reluctant to be judgmental about anyone.

"There's no telling what kind of upbringing someone like that has suffered through," he said about people who were cruel to him and to others. "I can't explain why I do what I do. Who am I to judge why someone else does what they do?" He shook his head sadly. "Who knows what makes someone do what they do?"

He had come to me because he was concerned that he had contracted a venereal disease. His bigger worry was that he might have passed it unknowingly along to his wife.

"I would just feel sick if I hurt her," he said with deep emotion.

As we spoke, John described his professional life to me. He had always worked long hours. A workaholic, he was as devoted to his career as he was to his family. His busy work schedule allowed him to easily hide his "secret life" from Maria. Twice a month he went with his friends to a special club for cross-dressers and transvestites. "I just tell Maria that I have a business engagement and would be home particularly late that evening.

"She never suspects anything," he said.

In spite of his freedom to engage in cross-dressing away from home, it had become more and more difficult for him to get dressed as a woman at home. One time, when he had expected his wife to be at work, he had gone home during lunch to try on some cosmetics and a dress he had bought for her. He had only just slipped on the dress when he was surprised by her early arrival home.

"My God!" she cried out, shocked and laughing at the

same time. "Have you gone completely crazy?"

Thinking fast, he said he was trying out a costume for an upcoming Mardi Gras. "I'd forgotten to mention it to you," he stammered. "Do you think I look too stupid like this?"

She studied him for a moment. Then, in an interestingly candid observation, she said, "You don't look bad actually." She nodded. "You would have been a very attractive woman." She kissed him on the cheek and then she left the room, going into the kitchen to make some coffee.

His heart pounding in his chest, he quickly got out of the dress and make-up. "I was in a complete faint the entire time," he told me. "Of course, I was still thrilled by her compliment," he added. When he joined her in the kitchen, she seemed to have already forgotten the incident.

She might have forgotten it—or, more likely, assigned it no importance—but that was not the case for him. That experience had convinced him never to get dressed up at home.

"Things were just safer for me at *Engagements*," he said, referring to the bar in Greenwich Village he frequented.

Not long before the afternoon when he was discovered by Maria, the bar had hosted a special "historical" evening. All the guests dressed up in elaborate costumes, each capturing a particular time in history. John chose to dress up as Marie Antoinette. He wore a pink dress with piles of lace. To complete the effect, he was attended by several servants.

"It was just marvelous," he said, finding a particular photograph in the envelope and showing it to me. "Beautiful, yes?"

Although fashion is hardly my area of expertise, I had to admit that the outfit and the overall effect were quite impressive. The sleeves of the dress were gorgeous.

To finish off the costume, he wore a dark wig and an elaborate hat topped with a heart and a pheasant feather.

His white shoes were detailed with pearls and diamonds.

"It was the most glorious moment of my life," he sighed. Then he looked me right in the eye. "I have the most incredible feelings when I dress up. These feelings are more sensual than sexual. They don't demand immediate and complete gratification like male-female sex does. It's as though every nerve in my body is alive.

"I don't even have to dress up to enjoy this feeling. I can experience it when I look at fashion magazines. Can you just imagine the beautiful things I buy for my wife? Transvestites *love* to shop for their wives." Then he sighed and lowered his eyes. "I've always tried to be so careful about the people I choose to have an affair with."

He raised his head and looked me sheepishly. He drew a deep breath. "About three weeks ago, I went to see a new movie at *Engagements*. During the movie, I suddenly became aware of someone's eyes on me. This sense of being absolutely undressed. Do you know that feeling? It is at once the most unsettling and the most wonderful sensation...

"Anyway, when I turned around, I looked directly into the eyes of this beautiful black man. Just magnificent. His head was shaven. He was muscular and obviously graceful. I later learned he was a belly dancer in the City.

"Well, when the movie was over, I went to change for the dance that was to begin later that evening. I have my own locker. I dressed in my usual—black skirt, black sweater, white high heels. After I was dressed, I came out to the dance floor.

I *felt* those eyes on me again. When I turned around, I saw him. He smiled and he came up to me." In a hushed voice that spoke of secrets and hidden things, he added, "He asked me to dance." He paused after that.

"I resisted at first. I told him I didn't like being with younger men... but he was persistent and so very attractive.

"We danced together and it was like we were created to be together. He moved so wonderfully."

John looked toward the window in my office. "Well, of course we ended up going to a room and laying on the bed. Have I already said that he had the most amazing body. His dick was huge. Like a banana. He put it in me deep, deep. I can't tell you how I felt with this young giant pounding away inside me. And then suddenly he finished, erupting like a volcano inside me. He was crying out how he loved me and that I was his beautiful woman.

"He took my penis in his mouth and I finished quickly. We hugged for a while. He called me his beautiful woman and I called him my hero.

"Later, after we dressed, we danced again to some beautiful romantic Italian songs." He shrugged. "Then I went home."

There was a moment of silence in the office. "My wife was already asleep when I got home." He smiled softly and toyed with the corner of the envelope. "Maria and I have never enjoyed a great sex life. I was happy to discover she didn't really like sex and I'm sure she was pleased that I never forced the issue.

"It worked out better. We were able to emphasize things we both enjoy—like good food and beautiful clothes.

"Anyway, the other day I realized I had blisters on my penis. I felt itchy all over my body. Especially my fingers and my ass. And my God, how I suffer at night. It's just terrible at night. My urine has become a deep yellow and I feel generally weak and achy.

"Maria and I haven't had sex for four months be we still sleep together in the same bed...

"Doctor," he pleaded, suddenly expressing an urgency he hadn't expressed before. "Please. You have to help me."

"I'll do everything I can," I assured him. "The first step is for us to diagnose what exactly it is that we're up against."

After a careful examination and lab work, I discovered that John suffered from scabies and hepatitis B, a viral disease contracted through sexual contact.

"Given the nature of this disease, I think you need to speak honestly with your wife," I told him when I shared the lab results with him.

He lowered his head. "I don't know how..."

"I'm sure it won't be easy but you it owe to her to tell her the truth. She might be sick herself."

As difficult as it was, John did confess to his wife. Her initial reaction was horror and anger. She demanded that they get a divorce. John described to me tears on both sides. "I could only imagine how she felt," he told me. "But I was desperate not to lose her. In spite of everything, I love her very much. And I love our life together..."

John begged her to try and work with him to find a way to make their marriage work.

"There was no way it was going to be a conventional marriage but then, it never was. Not really..."

Over the course of a couple of weeks, Maria struggled with John's confession of his sexual orientation.

"How could I not have known anything?" she asked me when she came in for an examination. "I *lived* with this man for twenty years..."

"Don't blame yourself," I said. "Your husband worked very hard at making sure you weren't aware of his secret. I believe he felt a great deal of shame regarding that aspect of your relationship, feeling he had to keep this important aspect of his personality from you."

Although she found it very difficult to accept that the man she had married and lived with for twenty years, the man who was the father of their two children, was a transvestite, she ultimately decided not to seek divorce.

"He's my best friend and the father of my children. I can't imagine what my life would be without him," she admitted. "Not that all this still doesn't shake me up every single morning..."

Her examination and lab work discovered that she too suffered from scabies and hepatitis B. Both John and Maria were successfully treated for their physical conditions but, as you might imagine, both their lives were changed profoundly. Although John was relieved to no longer have to hide his true nature from Maria, he felt a terrible sense of loss about the alteration in their marriage.

"I know I'm a deviate," John said to me when I last saw him. When he spoke, he had real bitterness in his voice. "But I can't live any other way. Maria would like me to simply *get better*. But I can't just *get better*. Besides, even if I could I don't even know if I want to, not really."

John continues to commute to the City from his upper-middle class, suburban home every day. Every day he stands on the train platform alongside hundreds of other commuters. He is dressed in his conservative business suits and carries his monogrammed briefcase.

No one on the platform, not a single one of his neighbors or friends, would suspect his secret life or the fact that he had suffered a serious STD.

It really can happen to anyone.

Sarah certainly learned that. So did Michael, the man she went with to the Cape. He felt awful about what had happened. Charm hadn't protected him from his loneliness when he separated from his wife nor did it shield him from his own need for sexual contact. It hadn't protected Sarah, whom he genuinely cared for. Neither of them saw themselves as vulnerable to sexually transmitted diseases. Even John, who was much more sexually promiscuous, never thought of himself as vulnerable.

But he was vulnerable. Each one of them ended up discovering just how vulnerable they really were.

Look at yourself in the mirror. Look at the people on the platform near you. Look at the people in your neighborhood. Look at the people in your office. Are they—or you—so much different from these three people?

If it can happen to the three of them, it really *can* happen to anyone.

The best protection against STD's is awareness and knowledge. A good dose of understanding would help as well.

As Sarah learned, STD's do happen to all sorts of people.

They happened to her.

And, as she would be the first to tell you, they can happen to you.

3

God's Scourge?

Often, in the midmorning, if my caseload is not too great, I will go for a walk outside the hospital. Depending on how much time I have—and the weather—I might walk a number of blocks.

On this particular day, I decided to walk toward the nearby college campus. There is just something about the atmosphere of a college that makes me feel very comfortable and pleased. Maybe my own college experience. I certainly enjoyed college.

It was while working as a volunteer in my college's infirmary that I first had an inkling about the future course of my career. I had wanted to be a doctor since I was a young boy but when I entered college I thought I might want to be a surgeon. However, during a slow evening at the infirmary one of the nurses, an older woman with graying hair and about ten pounds more than she would have liked, who was whose responsibility it was to facilitate the sex education seminars in the dormitories, asked me to help her.

"John, who is scheduled for this evening, has the flu and I need someone to help."

"Sure," I said.

We went over the material and, a short while later, we headed to one of the dormitories.

There were about thirty kids there. The presentation began with a survey and questionnaire. While the nurse spoke, I was compiling the data we learned from the surveys. During the presentation, there were a handful of joking comments and a few instances of embarrassed laughter but for the most part, everyone listened. Margaret didn't pull any punches. She talked professionally but in a straightforward, unblushing manner about the subject, surprising a lot of the students who must have expected something different from a woman who looked as if she could easily have been one of their mothers.

When she was finished, rather than ask for questions, we distributed index cards to everyone and asked that questions be written down. As she explained to me later, that was so no one would fail to ask a question due to embarrassment. When the cards were collected, the nurse went through each one, patiently and completely answering each question, even the ones that seemed to have been asked as a joke.

"Doesn't it hurt when someone has anal intercourse?" she read from one card.

In the back of the room there was noisily whispered, "All rights!" and some "Give me five!"

She smiled. "Good question," she said, quieting everyone immediately with her comfortable and direct manner. "You know, it's interesting. Every time I speak to a group of students, there is always a couple of `joke' questions. But sometimes, they're the most interesting.

"We tend to make jokes about the things we are most frightened of," she went on, explaining the incidence of "gallows humor" in the hospital. "Sex is like that. It confuses us. A lot of us feel that we're practiced at our sexuality..." she lifted the stack of questionnaires, "...although a much smaller number than you might think. But the fact of the matter is, sexuality calls into question a lot about ourselves, our upbringing, our hopes and our fears.

"We are ignorant about a great deal about sex and that is why we're here. What you don't know about sex *can* hurt you. Sexually transmitted diseases. Unwanted pregnancies. Emotional scarring. We can prevent a great deal of these unfortunate outcomes with one very important tool—knowledge.

"Safe sex does not mean no sex. It means knowledgeable, responsible—and hopefully enjoyable—sex."

Everyone was very attentive for the remainder of the presentation. Margaret answered the question about anal intercourse, making it clear that anal intercourse was *not* just an aspect of male homosexual behavior but that it was a part of lovemaking for many heterosexual couples as well.

"Sex should not hurt," Margaret said in conclusion. "Even if you derive some sexual pleasure from pain, that pain should not hurt in the way I'm using the word. No one should be forced to engage in sexual activity that they are uncomfortable with..."

When we returned to the infirmary, Margaret asked me how I thought it went.

"Pretty well," I said. "Everyone had their questions answered."

Margaret sighed. "I just hope we did some good. You know that a large percentage of the student visits we have are for something having to do with sexuality? Either for prevention or the treatment of sexual transmitted disease..."

The more I listened, the more I was convinced that I wanted to be a physician that dealt with people and their sexuality.

I often thought of Margaret during my walks to the college campus. In addition to her wonderful gifts as a facilitator of student groups, she had one gift that made her perfect for the role she played at the school. She was one hundred percent non-judgmental.

"It might not be what I do but that doesn't make it wrong," she told me once. "No, the only time I think someone does something that is wrong is if they hurt someone else. That's the line. No hurting."

I was thinking of Margaret when I came to the college campus near the hospital. Being such a lovely day, it was bustling with students and vendors. I loved the colors and the sounds and the smells. Glancing at my watch, I realized I still had a little bit of time so I allowed myself to wander further onto campus.Not far from the main quad, I found a man, a preacher, standing in the middle of students streaming by. He had propped up a large sign next to him. It read: AIDS IS GOD'S MESSAGE TO HOMOSEXUALS.

In addition to the sign, he was ranting and raving about how God was punishing sexually promiscuous people with all manners of disease. "The Book says it all!" he cried out. "Says it right here. Read it and learn! Read it and be saved!

"God tells you all! Right here in the Book of Deuteronomy.... the Lord will smite you with the boils of Egypt, and with the ulcers and the scurvy and the itch, of which you cannot be healed. you cannot be healed. The Lord will smite you with madness and blindness and confusion of mind; and you shall grope in darkness, and you shall not prosper in your ways...

"Does that not describe your suffering?" he cried out.

I listened for several moments, a rage beginning to boil within me. This man, with his religious certainty, was everything that Margaret had not been. He, and his beliefs, went a long way toward creating the kind of sexual mores which result in people hiding from their sexuality and, as a result, engaging in practices which are unsafe to them and to others.

He was so wrong. So damaging. Sexually transmitted diseases were not the scourge of God but the result of ignorance. They could be avoided—they *can* be. And most of them can be treated.

Whether viewed with the religious fervor of a Biblical curse or treated with the clinical formality of an epidemiologist, the reality is that sexual relations—gratifying and pleasurable—too often result in something other than pleasure. Too often they result in the contraction of an infectious disease.

Just ten or twenty years ago, the significance of sexually transmitted diseases (STD's) was cruelly underestimated by the general population. Called "venereal disease" then—after "Venus", the goddess of love, because of the Victorians' squeamishness at the mere mention of "sex" or "sexuality"—there was the erroneous belief that STD's would always be easily treatable with antibiotics, rendering them more like annoyances than real health threats.

Unfortunately, time and experience have brought home the error of that view. None of us can afford the luxury of ignorance when confronted by the threats posed by such sexually transmitted diseases as AIDS and herpes. Indeed, our single most potent weapon to counter the steady rise of these diseases is knowledge.

Several factors have conspired to foster an environment in which the number of STD's could increase. As families and society in general become less structured, the traditional restraints on sexual activity diminish. We are bombarded with an ethos that demands instant gratification, demands that play into the uncertainties of adolescence—a time of physical, physiological, and psychological change. Ignorance about sexual health and disease is coupled with the availability of new forms of contraception, forms which have essentially eliminated the *fear* of unwanted pregnancy (and its subsequent inhibition of sexual activity), though not the *reality* of it.

While the fundamental changes that are occurring in society are extremely difficult to address, we can and must certainly address the issue of ignorance when it comes to sexual health and STD's. To begin, we must address some misconceptions. These diseases exist at *all levels of society*, from the stars of entertainment and industry to the poor and indigent. STD's are not a poor man's disease. Infections cross all lines of age, education, income level, and ethnicity. The danger of contracting these diseases comes not from dirty toilet seats or casual contact but from *intimate, sexual contact*. Indeed, the single greatest risk factor in contracting STD's is having multiple sexual partners. STD's can be transmitted in the absence of traditional, genital-genital sexual intercourse. STD's can be contracted "the first time". As we shall see, STD's are often asymptomatic. However, the lack of symptoms does not provide protection. STD's can result in impairment of sexual organs, sometimes resulting in sterility or even death. Finally, although we have begun to hear and learn more and more about AIDS many other STD's continue to plague us.

Before STD's can be eradicated, ignorance regarding them must be eradicated. Ultimately, knowledge about STD's must also be a call to action—regarding personal sexual activity as well as public health policy.

However, I did not engage him in an argument. Not then and there. My battlefield was not the campus, not on that day, not with the glorious sun shining. My battlefield was in the hospital with my patients.

And, glancing at my watch, it was there that I had to return.

I looked back one last time at the preacher preaching his message and I shook my head. Perhaps he was well-meaning but the end result of his rigid judgments was that people were suffering. It seemed to me to be a terrible shame.

4

Symptoms?

While it might seem a bit odd to say it, Sarah was lucky. Although she contracted an STD, she was fortunate enough to suffer symptoms that prompted her to seek medical care. Far too often, STD's remain symptomless. When they do, they become silent terrorists wreaking havoc on your body.

Gonorrhea is the oldest of all sexual diseases. In addition, it is also the most prevalent. In 1986, there were more than 896,000 cases reported in the United States. However, many cases go unreported and estimates suggest that as many as two million cases occur annually. In the 1950s, public health officials believed that the use of penicillin had effectively eliminated gonorrhea. Clearly, they were wrong.

Gonorrhea is caused by the bacterium *Neisseria gonorrheae* or *gonococcus*. Because this bacterium flourishes in mucous membranes, the moist protective coat that lines all orifices of the body, sexual activity (whether oral-vaginal, oral-anal, penile-anal, oral-penile, oral-oral, or genital-genital) provides a fertile haven for the bacterium.

"Which explains the sores I received in my mouth," Sarah noted.

"That is correct. Although many people presume that STD's can only be caught through traditional genital-genital intercourse, every one of the body's orifices are wonderful hosts to STD's."

While every body orifice represents a host area, most cases of gonorrhea result from genital-genital intercourse. As a consequence, because of the much larger surface area of the mucous lining of the vagina, women have a much greater risk of contracting gonorrhea than men do. In spite of this, and quite ironically, men are much more likely to suffer the symptoms of gonorrhea. *As many as eighty percent of women* who contract gonorrhea exhibit no symptoms. In fact, most women do not know they have a gonorrheal infection unless their infected partner tells them or unless they happen to have a smear and culture taken during a routine gynecological exam. This alone should encourage sexually active women to seek testing for gonorrhea during their regular check-ups.

"So, in a curious way, I was very fortunate to have suffered as I did," Sarah said.

"Yes. As we will come to learn, even when STD's are treatable, unless addressed early they can result in pelvic inflammatory disease (PID). PID is one of the most common causes of infertility in women of childbearing age."

Although as many as forty percent of men with gonorrhea are asymptomatic, those who do exhibit symptoms do so within two to ten days after contact. In men, the urethra and the rectum are the most likely sites of infection. Generally, symptoms include the sudden onset of frequent, painful urination as well as a purulent (pus-like) discharge from the urethra.

In the absence of treatment, the infection will spread into the genitourinary tract within two to three weeks, affecting the posterior urethra, the prostate, the seminal vesicles, and the epididymis. Infection in the prostate is accompanied by pelvic tenderness and pain, fever and difficulty in urination. If the epididymis becomes inflamed, there is a feeling of heaviness in the affected testicle, and inflammation of the scrotal skin. If the infection spreads to the other testicle, infertility is a real possibility.

The primary infection site for women is the cervix. Again, because the vast majority of women are asymptomatic, there is the increased danger of complications, resulting in pelvic inflammatory disease (PID). Within two months, the untreated gonococcal organisms infect the internal reproductive organs and pelvic cavity. During menstruation and immediately following, the organisms travel rapidly, causing painful intercourse, nonmenstrual uterine bleeding and the inflammation of the fallopian tubes. As the body tries to "wall off" the infection, scarring of the tubes frequently occurs, with infertility a possible result.

While these are the primary sites of infection and their possible subsequent complications, the gonococcus can also enter the blood stream and travel to the joints, resulting in gonococcal arthritis. It may even travel to the heart valves.

Other sites for nongenital infection include the mouth and throat, the anus and the rectum, and the eyes. During oral intercourse, the gonococcus can invade the throat (this is less of a threat during cunnilingus than fellatio). Rectal gonorrhea results from anal intercourse and so affects women in heterosexual relations although more commonly men in homosexual relations. The incidence of gonorrhea in the eyes is minimal in adults, usually resulting when they touch their genitals and then transfer the infected pus to their eyes. The primary danger of gonorrhea to the eyes is to newborn infants, transferred from the mother's cervix to their eyes during birth.

The diagnosis of gonorrhea requires a culture of discharges taken from the affected body sites. For men, this usually means a sample of the discharge coming from the urethra. In women, this generally requires a sample taken from the cervix. Although the procedure to accomplish this is sometimes uncomfortable, it is rarely painful. A cotton-tipped swab is inserted into the cervix to retrieve a sample of the discharge. However, in cases of gonorrhea in both men and women, cultures can be taken from discharge at other body sites, including the throat, rectum, or vagina itself.

Unfortunately, at this time there exists no satisfactory blood test for gonorrhea as there is for a number of other STD's. If there were then routine screening could be done permitting diagnosis in those people who are asymptomatic.

"But there *is* a standard treatment for gonorrhea," Sarah said, prompting an answer she already knew.

"Yes, there is. A fairly effective treatment. However, as with many treatments, we have to be concerned that there will develop resistant diseases and so we must emphasize that prevention is much more important than treatment."

5

PROTECT YOURSELF! BUT HOW?

During my walk back to the hospital, I couldn't shake the image of the angry preacher from my thoughts. With his flaming red hair and flared nostrils, he was the physical embodiment of "fire and brimstone." His message was troubling to me because, while the religion he pretended to represent taught love and forgiveness he preached anything but those lofty things.

Even so, there was one word in his angry diatribe he kept returning to which also continued to play in my mind—truth.

As I thought about it, I considered my patient, John. He had professed—and I believed him—to be sincere in his love for his wife. Yet, he was not honest with her, was not "truthful" with her until he was forced to be.

Or was he?

The whole notion of love and sex, the way our culture and society has presented it to us—foisted it upon us—nearly guarantees that the two will come into conflict. One, love, is the foundation of our basic social institution—marriage. And here

I do not necessarily mean a marriage sanctioned by a particular religious institution or civil convention but rather the commitment between two people to establish a life-long relationship. Sex, on the other hand, is very often the response to a primal urge that can be as transitory as a rushed episode between two people who never exchange their names.

Our social convention expects, demands, that the two co-join. Reality intervenes a tremendous amount of the time.

One of my patients, a homosexual, suggested that the gay community had a better sense of a reasonable relationship between sex and love. Because the gay community tends to be so promiscuous monogamy has never been the basis for a long-term relationship.

Of course, the rampant promiscuity was more evident before the AIDS epidemic hit.

However, the basic position is an interesting one. Why do we insist (at least theoretically) on monogamy in our relationships? Statistics suggest that a large majority of people is unsuccessful in maintaining monogamy. The divorce rate speaks to the same reality.

And, as a result, honesty suffers.

John considered Maria his best friend as well as his wife and yet he was forced—by convention—to hide from her one of the most basic aspects of who he was.

The Preacher can condemn him. The Preacher can demand that we look to truth. But the reality is for most people it is impossible to make their sexual selves and their conventional selves seamless. As a result, there are furtive, illicit sexual encounters, encounters that too often result in disease.

To many people, there are only two venereal (love) diseases—syphilis and gonorrhea. The reality is that there are many other diseases that can be spread through sexual contact, including herpes, Chlamydia, venereal warts, vaginitis, hepatitis B and AIDS.

One cruel aspect of some of these diseases is that they present without symptoms in too many people, leading to ever more serious conditions. Without treatment, these diseases can lead to major health problems such as sterility, blindness, insanity, heart disease and even death.

Fortunately, there are ways to reduce the risk of getting an STD. You can:

have only one sex partner, whose health is known;

use a condom with a spermicide during sex;

urinate after sex;

wash after sex;

don't have sex with a person who shoots drugs or who ever did;

don't have anal sex.

No one can tell by "looking" if a person is infected with an STD. "Truth" as we know, is one of the first casualties of sexual episodes.

Protect yourself!

6

MORE PATIENTS

When I returned to the hospital, I stopped to wash my hands. The receptionist informed me that my next patient was waiting to see me. As I finished drying my hands I asked that the patient be sent to my office.

"Hello," I said, extending my hand to an attractive, young woman. "Please come in."

Chloe was dressed in jeans and a pink tee shirt with lace at the collar. Her blonde hair was cut short. She wore heavy mascara and lipstick. Her skin had a handful of old acne scars. Her eyes, brown, were clear.

"I.. I don't know how to start," she said softly.

I smiled. "Why not start at the beginning?" I suggested.

She shrugged. "I feel pretty stupid," she said, looking down at her hands.

"Why don't we begin with what's bothering you today. Why did you come in to see me?"

"I've got stuff... discharge.. you know.. down there," she said, nodding down toward her lap.

I asked Chloe some basic health questions before returning to the discharge she was concerned with. She was clearly ill at ease and the first thing I needed to do was to make her feel a bit more comfortable and safe.

When she seemed to be relaxing a bit, I asked her when she first noticed the discharge.

"Only a few days ago," she said. Then she crossed her arms. "It all started at that damned party..."

Her story begins in the taxi on the way home from a party where she and her boyfriend, Raymond, had both been drinking heavily.

"I'd say I was drunk," Chloe told me. "But I wasn't any more drunk than Raymond was. He almost gave the driver the wrong address of my apartment. When we finally got upstairs to my apartment my dog, Nelson, started to lick my face. Raymond laughed and said it was because the dog liked the taste of the whiskey on my lips. I told Raymond it was because my dog loved me.

"God, I was *so* drunk. The room was spinning. Raymond teased me that if I loved Nelson so much I should go to bed with him."

"You'd like that, wouldn't you?" I challenged him. You know, I was so drunk I was almost considering it—just to get at Raymond. He was really starting to annoy me.

"I got out of my dress and my underwear and just collapsed back on my mattress. My legs were bent off the side of the bed and the cool breeze coming in through the windows felt good on my tits and my vagina.

"I felt myself drifting off to sleep when I felt something warm and wet between my legs. It felt so good. I love having my clit licked and being lost in that space right before sleep made the feeling even more intense.

"I could hear myself moaning. I was pinching my nipples and just enjoying all the sensations.

"Then the licking stopped and I felt a hard prick stabbing between my legs. Ah, it was so good when it found its way into my vagina. My legs were out of control. They were spasming all over the place. Deeper and deeper. Over and over. I was going over the edge myself. I remember crying out with this intense orgasm and then feeling globs of sperm explode inside of me. So warm and nice.

"I must have fallen asleep because a while later I opened my eyes and there was Nelson standing over me, panting with his tongue hanging out.

"I looked over at the corner of the room and Raymond was there sleeping peacefully on the floor. I reached down between my legs. There was still thick sperm in my vagina so I wasn't dreaming but who—or what—did I have sex with? Raymond or Nelson?

"I couldn't believe it. I wasn't sure. I mean, I couldn't imagine getting fucked by my dog but... it was just too weird. But I was *so* drunk. And I had heard of weirder things happening.

"This girl I know, when she was tripping on acid, she ended up in some elevator with three guys and another girl. She didn't remember getting there or anything...

"Anyway, two weeks later there was a funny—not funny ha ha but funny strange—discharge coming from my vagina. There were stains on my underwear and it burned when I peed.

"I was so scared. I hadn't ever had anything like that before. I was ready to kill Raymond but he swore to me that hadn't fucked around with anyone else. He took out his penis to show me. `See', he said. `I got nothing on it.' He didn't either."

"I think we should examine you and find out exactly what's going on with your body," I said. "My nurse will take you to an examination room."

My examination of Chloe indicated that the discharge she had noticed. I took a culture and then explained to her that, although I would have to wait for the test results, her symptoms and her physical presentation indicated that she likely had contracted gonorrhea.

"From my fucking dog?" she cried out.

Not knowing exactly how to respond to that, I remained silent.

"I swear, I'm gonna kill that Raymond. If I find out that he's been whoring around..."

"Why don't we wait and see what the test results tell us," I counseled. "If there is something that needs to be discussed, perhaps we can have Raymond come in."

"Oh yeh, he'll come in all right...."

Sitting in my office, I had no doubt that Chloe had contracted gonorrhea. My problem was what to make of the story she had told me. Certainly she had had too much to drink the evening that she had related to me. But the story about her dog?

While there was the tendency to be dismissive about such events, my own

experience with patients has made me very reluctant to doubt even the most outlandish sounding story. When it comes to sexuality and sexual behavior, there really is very little that falls within the parameters of "normal."

It happens that the national discourse at this moment

involves the sexual relations between the President of the United States and an intern working in the White House. Of course, given my profession, this discourse interests me greatly. Not because of the so-called "impeachable offenses". I cannot comment on these. No, the secrecy and subsequent "misinformation" that may or may not have been given concerning this affair is the nature of the relations that are being considered.

For most of my patients, the exact nature of how they contracted a sexually transmitted disease is not information that they would like to be known publicly. Even those who are not involved in "adulterous" affairs are not anxious—this is an understatement—to have their sexual history known by their friends, family, co-workers or, for that matter, strangers.

It is difficult for them to confess the details of their relations to me—and many choose not to. Many of my patients prefer to come to me with their physical symptoms and have me try to heal their bodies. They do not want me to know any more about them than what their diseases tell me.

So, the desired secrecy of this affair is of little interest to me. What I do find interesting is the perceived notion of what is "perverse". In this regard, the President's cigar seems to have gotten a fair amount of attention. Indeed, among certain populations the issue of oral sex is an issue of perversion. Why, there are still states in the Union which count sodomy (which includes oral sex) as a crime—even when engaged in by consenting adults. These adults may even be married... to one another!

Perversion.

We seem to find perversion in any behavior which we do not comfortably engage in. This perception—and rush to judgment—defines sexual mores in any culture. However, the truth is, the sex drive is so basic and so powerful that humans will almost always find a means to fulfill it. When a society or circumstances makes the fulfillment of the sex drive difficult then the individual will go to great lengths to find fulfillment.

Hence, "illicit" sex.

But, when examined objectively, what is so unusual about inserting a phallic object into a vagina? How many "normal" girls and women—some matronly and even members of your church group—do so?

That voice that cries perversion, that voice that in my mind echoes the red-haired preacher, does so much damage.

A person can no more deny sexual appetite than the desire—the need—for food. Should food be denied or, to push the analogy, the exact same food be served meal after meal, day after day, week after week... you would not be surprised to find that people would d all sorts of things to acquire food. They would plant it, barter for it, steal it... whatever.

So too with sex.

So, while it may seem that Chloe's question as to whether she might have gotten gonorrhea from her dog is a bit startling at first flush, it is not something that I would ever sit in judgment of.

However, as it turned out, whether it is possible or not, Chloe did not get her STD from her dog.

When the definite diagnosis was made, I contacted Chloe to come in and urged her to have Raymond come in as well.

"If you are sexually active with your boyfriend and you have an STD there is a strong likelihood that he will have it as well," I said when she protested.

"That son of a..." she muttered. "If he gave this to me..."

But once again, Chloe was on the wrong course. It turned

out that Raymond did *not* have gonorrhea.

"I told you I was clean," Raymond said to Chloe. Then he narrowed his eyes at her. "What gives?"

Chloe hung her head. Slowly, the real story came out, one that had nothing to do with anything particularly strange or unusual about her sex life. She invented the story about being drunk and worrying about having sex with her dog. And, Raymond had been telling the truth as well.

Chloe herself was the source of the STD. She had contracted gonorrhea from a one-night stand which she'd had with a man she met in a bar. In short, a story as old as time itself.

If Chloe was willing to go to great lengths to concoct a story about how she might have gotten an STD, a patient I saw the following week was very clear about how he'd gotten sick.

Francis, a bright, young assistant physics professor was the last person you would suspect of STD's. At twenty-four, he still looked like the virgin he had been only a year or so earlier. He was just a shade overweight and had the look of a very good student who spent more time with books than with other people.

"Doc," he said to me when he first visited my office, "I was plain scared of women. The thought of calling a girl up and asking her for a date filled me with such dread that I would get physically ill."

Francis was so convinced of his own "unworthiness" that he sank deeper and deeper into his studies. When he did think about his social life—or lack of one—he felt depressed. He was convinced that he was doomed to live out his life as a virgin.

He might very well have lived to suffer that fate but for the appearance of an old friend of his—John. John had been an acquaintance of Francis' since high school where they had played some sports together and worked on several projects for classes.

While Francis was a bit overweight even then—and not particularly athletic—John was active, well-built and aggressive. He was everything Francis seemed not to be. While Francis was afraid to even talk about girls John would brag that he was going to grow up to produce pornography when he was older.

So intent was he on realizing this goal that he tried to get a girl in school so drunk that she would undress for the camera but before he could actually get the camera rolling, she realized what was really going on and she rushed away.

After high school, Francis and John went their separate ways—Francis to college and then to a job in a small college. John off to California. Francis was both surprised and pleased to receive a call from John.

"Hey, Francis. How are you?"

"Good, good," Francis replied, stunned by the sound of John's voice. It seemed as if all the years since high school simply vanished.

"Listen, I'm only in town for a few days. How about meeting for drinks?"

"Great!"

Over drinks, they caught up with one another's lives since they'd last seen one another. Francis was not surprised to learn that John had, in fact, realized his dream and had become a producer of pornographic films in California.

"I guess the arcs of our lives haven't changed at all," Francis said, suddenly dejected. "I'm still the virginal loser I was back in high school."

John studied his old friend over the rim of his wine glass.

"Look, I think I can help you," he said simply.

Before the evening was out, John had invited Francis to visit his home in San Diego. "We'll have a great time," John promised.

Francis went to California early the following month. John met him at the airport and then drove him to his home where they arrived to find a party in full swing.

"You had to see it," Francis said, shaking his head as if he was still worried he'd been dreaming. "There were gorgeous women *everywhere*! They all looked like models."

Some of the women were drinking. A handful were swimming in the pool. A group were gathered around John, who hardly seemed to mind the attention.

"Francis! Francis!" John called, bringing his old friend over. "Come here, there's someone I want you to meet."

John introduced Francis to Sandy, a blonde and very sexy young woman. Sandy was dressed in a short tee shirt and cut-off jeans. When she smiled at Francis she displayed the most beautiful teeth he'd ever seen. He didn't know where to look first. Her face. Her magnificent body. Her smile... He was dizzy with her beauty.

Sandy said that she was an actress. "Why don't we sit down and talk?" she said, guiding him toward a couch in the living room.

She was so beautiful and sexy the way she crossed and uncrossed her legs that Francis quickly got an erection. He felt himself blushing when Sandy smiled again.

"How flattering," she said, reaching out and closing her hand around the lump in his trousers.

She massaged his erection for a couple of moments before running her tongue over her lips. "I'm feeling awfully horny myself," she confessed, getting up and leading him to a bedroom.

Once inside the bedroom, Sandy slipped down to her knees in front of Francis. On her way down, she had taken off his trousers and underwear. "Umm, nice," she said, examining his penis. Then she slipped it into her mouth.

Francis could not remember experiencing such pleasure before. The suction of her hot, moist mouth. Her hands on his ass. He thought he would explode then and there. But she was too practiced to allow that to happen.

She got up a moment later and began taking off her clothes. Francis could only stand there, his erect penis sticking straight out, his trousers around his feet, and stare at her. Sandy was quickly naked. She had been wearing no underwear under her clothes.

"What are you waiting for?" she asked with a teasing giggle. She jumped on the bed.

Francis threw off his clothes and joined her. Anxious though he was, she took complete control for setting the pace. Sandy pushed him back and then mounted him, riding his dick as if she was riding a horse.

"Oh God, umm, oh, oh..." She sounded just like the actresses in the porno films that he had seen. "Your dick is so nice and hard. I love the way it feels. Oh, I love it, love it..."

She came several times, screaming out in pleasure each time. And then Francis experienced the one thing he had longed to experience since he had reached adolescence—he came inside a beautiful woman.

"Thanks to John, I had become a man," was the way he described it to me.

After his visit to California, he had no trouble meeting a

nurse from a local hospital.

"We hit it off right away," he said. "We were naked in bed that first night. But, about six months later, I began to feel weak. Like I had the flu or something. I had enlarged lymph nodes and a rash in my mouth.

"When I went to the doctor, he said I had a yeast infection in my mouth. At about the same time, I noticed a white rash on my penis..."

One thing about my patients, they give a human face to sexually transmitted diseases. Their passions are so real. But, as I've said, sexual passion—sexual behavior—is an inborn drive in human beings. Even infants show signs of sexual behavior. Of course, the sex drive can be modified by culture, society and interpersonal realities.

In America there is tremendous pressure to control sexuality. But, if there is one thing I have learned through my life and my medical practice it is that sexuality cannot be cut off. People *need* to be sexual creatures.

So, what about Francis? What disease did he suffer from? He seemed like a very nice young man, a sympathetic young man. But that didn't protect him from STD's any more than charm had protected Sarah and Michael.

My examination resulted in a diagnosis of candidiasis and HIV. No doubt he acquired the HIV virus from his one-night with the porn star, Sandy. His HIV developed into full-blown AIDS.

Several months after he first came to me, Francis was dead.

His "reward" for finally losing his virginity was his mortality.

Innocence is no protection either.

The most difficult aspect of treating diseases of any kind is remembering that behind every disease is a very human being who is suffering. My patients put a human face on STD's. However, to put a human face on STD's one need look no further than their mirror. *We* are all the human face of STD's.

7:

SOME FACTS AND FALLACIES ABOUT STD'S

One of my patients once responded to his diagnosis by claiming, "But I only had sex with this married woman. Her husband didn't fool around. She was clean..." He hung his head. "Or so I thought.

"I guess I should have known from my own experience that she did."

Taking someone's word regarding their health is not enough. Nor is it possible to tell if someone has an STD because they are not "clean". You can't even be sure even if you know that your potential partner is not sexually promiscuous. You don't even have to have sexual contact with someone to acquire an STD. Syphilis and HIV can be transmitted by blood.

It is quite understandable that, given the intimate nature of STD's, that individuals being tested for them be anxious regarding confidentiality. In the case of HIV not only do patients have to contend with the dread and anxiety associated with the disease itself but they must also fear possible discrimination if they are found to be positive.

As a physician who treats STD's, I spend a great deal of time with each of my patients, promoting candor and trust. I always speak with my patients in my office before conducting a physical examination. I want them to be comfortable and be able to share with me the experiences that have contributed to their illness.

It is very important that patients suffering from an STD not be judged for their actions, behavior or decisions. As we have noted, we are all sexual animals. That is a reality of our nature. How we express our sexuality is a matter of great individuality. Being judgmental cannot aid in the healing of any individual suffering from an STD.

Examination, diagnosis and treatment of such illnesses is often painful. It is always embarrassing. No one is happy to have to share intimate details of their lives—especially details which open bare behavior which they might be ashamed of in retrospect. "Shoulds" and "should nots" have no place in the treatment of patients with STD's. Promiscuity, homosexuality, deviations from the "norm"—these are all activities and behaviors which must be accepted by any physician treating patients with STD's.

Just as the physician must be non-judgmental in treating a patient with an STD, the patient must be honest with the physician.

Often, my patients come to me with misconceptions about STD's which must be dispelled if they are to avoid another infection in the future. I have heard every sort of explanation, excuse, expression of denial and misconception that you can imagine. Just a brief sampling of the many things I have heard will give you a clear idea:

I know exactly where I got this disease;

I got this disease from the last person I had sex with;

when my symptoms are gone, my infection will be cured;

I know I got this infection from someone who was dirty;

my symptoms are not from an STD's but from some other cause—like stress, chemical burns, zipper trauma, menstrual cramping...;

if I don't have any symptoms, I'm okay;

my symptoms, if and when they appear, will be unambiguous;

STD's do not lead to serious complications;

STD's are not transmitted through any other method than genital-genital sexual intercourse;

STD's cannot be prevented;

I can share my medication or discontinue my medication;

STD's are related to social status and personal cleanliness;

birth control pills prevent V.D. (In fact, birth control pills induce chemical changes in the vaginal secretions which promotes an environment that actually *encourages* the growth of organisms that cause STD's.)

These alone should be enough to indicate the degree of misinformation on the street and in the minds of too many people. Underscoring all these is the most basic of misconceptions, the misconception that we have addressed several times already—it can't happen to *me.*

It can happen to you. It can happen to your spouse, to your neighbors or to your friends. Remember, the same sex drive that occupies your thoughts and behavior does the same for everyone else. Sigmund Freud believed that sexual energy along with hostility and aggression accounted for the motivation behind most human behavior. While a great many people have disagreed with Freud's teachings I have yet to hear someone present a convincing argument that suggests that the basic drives we have as humans do not include the sex drive.

In other words, sex drives us all. As I noted early on, we may deny our sex drive or we may embrace it. Either way, our actions and behaviors are a response to that drive.

For most of us, our behavior represents some synthesis of both extremes.

In 1970, there were approximately 42 million sexually active people between the ages of 15 and 34 in America. In 1992, that number jumped to 82 million. More and more female teenagers and single adults are initiating sexual activity at earlier ages. In addition, single people are remaining single—and sexually active—for longer periods of time.

To put a human face on these numbers—your daughter is likely to be engaging in sexual activity as early as her freshman year in high school. The young woman—and not so young woman—working in your office is likely to be engaging in regular sexual activity with different partners.

The same is true for teenage boys and single men.

The rise in premarital sex which has been occurring since the turn of the century jumped markedly with the easy availability of birth control pill, the development and growth of the women's liberation movement and social conditions and ideologies which promoted later marriages, women's entry into the labor force and a high divorce rate.

The increase in the divorce rate brought with it several relevant consequences. Because divorced men and women tend to be more sexually active than sexually experienced newlyweds—and engage in sexual activity with multiple partners—they are particularly vulnerable to STD's.

"I guess I fall into that demographic pretty well," Sarah

had noted ruefully when I shared these numbers with her.

"Statistics are statistics," I reminded her. "Individuals are always individuals. Each of my patients is an individual with his or her own particular history and story.

"As for divorced men and women, while it is true that their sexual activity makes them vulnerable to STD's, the reality is that many marriages are anything but monogamous to begin with and, as a result, there is the risk of STD's in those situations as well."

Once again, for all the demographic, social or economic changes, the bottom line is represented by one simple fact which constantly presents itself—we are all at risk for contracting STD's.

Regardless of any other understanding of STD's that must be our starting point. And, once we accept that fact, we are in a much better place to learn about STD's.

8

A Reflection

How many times have I come home after seeing three or four patients who have poured out stories of sexual intimacies that have led to STD's and entered a world which seems to render my hospital experience surreal.

Like everyone else in my neighborhood, I return home in the evening and my wife greets me.

"How was your day?" she might ask.

How was my day? Do I tell her the truth? Do I tell her about the young woman who, getting drunk at a frat party engages in sex with multiple partners—and ends up with an STD? Do I tell her about the young woman, married for only three years, who is frightened by her inability to become pregnant and finds out that her difficulty is the result of a sexually transmitted disease that she had contracted as a teenager but had never suffered any symptoms?

"The usual," is all I will generally reply.

Sometimes, in the evening, I will reflect on the apparent dichotomy of my life—my private life of comfort and my professional life filled with the confusion of disease, the result of often misplaced passion.

One evening when I was reflecting on this very aspect of my life, it occurred to me that my thoughts were true of everyone. Those I knew and those I did not.

The patients I saw at the hospital were both literally and figuratively stripped naked before me. Left without their protective clothing, they are easy to read, to judge, to misunderstand.

One of the criticisms often given to Freud was that he devised his psychology based on pathologies rather than on mentally healthy people. Certainly, the same could be said of me. I see patients whose sexuality results in disease. But in their private lives, clothed, they are certainly very different people. People with families. Friends. Dreams. Hopes.

And, by the same token, those people who we know primarily by how they would have us know them, by their dreams and hopes, are the same as my patients when stripped of their clothing—physical and figurative.

It occurs to me that the criticism of Freud is misplaced. We are all the same. We are as much defined by our so-called pathologies as we are by our so-called normalcy.

Never is that more true than when we consider our sexuality.

We brings me back to my wife's question. What *should* any of us say when we get home from work? Do we tell our wives or our husbands or our lovers the truth about the inner lives—and sometimes "outer lives"—we've lived that day in their absence?

Or should we simply move forward with the tacit understanding that some things are more appropriate kept to ourselves?

9

MORE CASES

Most patients come to me with some sadness or sense of remorse, if not about their behavior then certainly about the fact that they were suffering from a disease. Roberto came in fighting mad.

"Look, Doc," he demanded as soon as he had entered my office. "Look what that bitch did to me!" He was opening his trousers as he walked toward me. "I tried to calm her down... tell her to take it easy..."

I motioned to the door. Roberto paused long enough to return to the door and close it behind him. Then he strode back toward me. "Look at my dick, Doc."

Roberto, a tall, young Puerto Rican, stopped in front of me. His hand, shaking slightly, pulled down the zipper of his pants. "Just look at this, Doc!"

Before glancing at the penis is his hand, I quickly took in Roberto's physical presence. He was a tall, well-built young man with a pony-tail and smooth skin. He appeared to be in general good health.

When I looked at his penis, I could see the reason for his anger and discomfort. The end of his penis was red and there was a copious discharge.

"How long have you noticed the discharge?" I asked him.

He shrugged. "A few days."

"Zip up. Let's go into the examination room."

In the examination room, I discovered that, in addition to the irritation and discharge his also had an enlarged right testicle.

As I examined him, he continued to berate the woman again.

"Why don't you slow down and tell me what happened?" I asked as I continued my examination.

"Oh, I'll tell you what happened. I'll tell you for sure, Doc. Fuckin' bitch. I'll tell you the whole goddamned story..." His eyes flashed with fresh anger. His voice was sharp and clear. "Look, I was weary, you know. Things weren't workin' out for me at all.

"I didn't have no job—and I didn't have no hope of gettin' one right away. I was pissed and I figured the best thing for me to do was to chill a bit in the bar. Just relax and get my thoughts together.

"So I was sitting at the bar, drinkin' a beer... oh, did I tell you that my bitch of a girlfriend was screwin' around with some other guy? Well, you can bet that didn't improve my mood one bit.

"So I was just damned pissed and I wanted to have a cool beer to wash away some of the world's bullshit. You know how it is, don't you, Doc?"

I nodded my head as I took a culture of the discharge coming from his penis.

"All I wanted was to figure out some way to get enough money together to get my ass down to the Caribbean. Well, I was nursin' my bear, runnin' through all sorts of possibilities when I notice this guy come into the bar. The guy just stunk of money." Roberto shrugged. "Had to be about forty-five, I'd figure. Decent shape but other than that, pretty average.

"There was something about him that gave me the creeps. He didn't belong in the bar. He was wearing this real expensive suit, not a drug dealer's suit, a businessman's suit. I noticed when he ordered a beer he had a fine gold watch on his wrist.

"I noticed that all right. How do you think it made me feel, seein' this guy just oozin' money when all I could think about was how I didn't have none? And you know what made the whole thing worse? The dude kept on starin' at me. At me!

"I wasn't botherin' no one. I was nursin' my own beer and here was this dude who had no business bein' in the same bar as me sittin' there an' starin' at me. Woulda made my blood boil if it didn't make me so nervous.

"I was figurin' that the guy was a cop. Why not? Stranger shit's happened. I just got out of the can about six months ago an' I didn't want no trouble with no cops, that's for sure."

He shook his head as if he couldn't figure out how the fates had brought him to my office.

"I guess I shouldna hit my ex-girl but shit, she was fuckin' around on me. What the hell was I supposed to do? Ignore it? So I hit her a couple of times and she got me canned.

"But I did my time and came out all right. I wasn't botherin' no one and I wasn't breakin' no laws. So I couldn't figure what this guy wanted from me. And then he comes walking over to where I was sittin' and he asked if he could join me.

"Shit. What was I gonna say? No? I told him it was a free

country and he could sit wherever he wanted. So he smiled at me and sat down. I noticed this big diamond ring on his finger when he did.

"Jeez, I couldn't figure what kind of mess I was about to get myself into. Cops? Pinky rings? Hell, all I wanted was to make a few bucks and get my ass down to the Caribbean.

"Well, the way this guy keeps lookin' at me I figure he's no cop and he's no crook either. Now I'm nervous 'cause I figure him to be a faggot. I didn't want none of that shit so I told him straight out that I didn't like the way he was lookin' at me and if he was lookin' to get laid he could just move along somewheres else.

"Sonabitch laughed. Said, no no. He wasn't lookin' to get laid but he did have a deal for me if I was interested in makin' a few bucks. Well, he had my attention with that so I said, go on, I'm listenin'.

"He started tellin' me about this bitch he had that he wanted to get off his back. Said she was older than he was and he just couldn't get it up with her. He told me she sent him out looking for a young Latin guy who could fuck her real good. And, get this, she wanted him to watch while she was gettin' fucked.

"I'll tell ya, Doc, there's a lot of weird shit in this world.

"I was about to tell him that I didn't want any part of his weird-ass shit when he said it was worth an easy $200 an hour to me. You can guess how that registered with me. $200 an hour sounded like a million to me right then. I figured, what the hell? How bad could it be anyway? I told him, okay. I'd do it.

"He stuck his hand out and said his name was Carl. I got a shiver from his handshake. Limp and wet. I hate that. Anyway, he said let's go and he led me outside to his car. When I was gettin' in, he asked me if I wanted any dope. Hey, I don't mind a little weed now and then when I can get it so I said sure.

"I smoked some of a doobie as we drove to an apartment on 87th Street, not far from the park.

"When we got there, he took out some coke and we snorted that too. Now *that* was some pretty great dope. I'll tell you, Doc, when I got out of that damned car I felt like fuckin' superman.

"He asked me if I was ready to go up to the apartment and I told him sure. Doc, I never been in an apartment like this. Big. Beautiful. Marble all over the fuckin' place. A real rich guy's paradise.

"Carl took me into the den and we snorted some more coke. Then he led me into this room. There was only a small light on and it was covered with a lace cloth so the room was pretty dark. Took me a minute for my eyes to adjust. When they did, I saw this big bed covered with black sheets. This woman, hell, Doc, she had to be about sixty-five, was naked and tied face down to the bed posts with some stockings.

"God, she was so tiny and shriveled up. I felt weird, I'll tell you that. Carl said I should take off my clothes. I felt a lot weirder standin' there naked with Carl there and this shriveled up old lady tied up on the bed like that but, I was already pretty high and I was in it for the money, right?

"I stood by the bed and I asked the lady what her name was. She didn't answer me. That really pissed Carl off. He'd been nothin' but nice to me since I met him but now I saw another side of him. He took up a stick that was laying on the floor and he started to beat her on the ass with it.

"He yelled at her and told her to tell me her name. She said her name was Sabina. Then she called him Master.

"Weird shit." Roberto said, shaking his head. "Then Carl looked at me and told me to fuck her up the ass. So I did it while Carl sat in a chair and watched. When I was finished, he peeled off $200 and handed me a few damned good joints. I guess as a tip.

"After that, I was so wasted I could have fucked a dog.

"I figured it was all pretty easy and, after a couple of days, it was even somethin' I was jokin' about with people. But then, a few days after that, I was screamin' in pain when I tried to pee and my fuckin" balls felt like they were on fire." He pointed down at his crotch. "Look what that fuckin' bitch did to me!" he cried out.

I washed my hands at the sink in the examination room. "We'll know with certainty what you've gotten when the culture comes back. However, based on the symptoms you've described and my physical exam, I would say that you are likely suffering from gonorrhea complicated by epididinitis..."

"Epidid...?"

"Basically a very fancy word for inflamed testicles which results from a gonorrhea type bacterial infection."

"Can you help me, Doc?"

I smiled and nodded my head. "Yes, I believe I can."

Treating cases like Roberto's give me one of the few opportunities that I have to smile. For now—and, given the threat of resistant strains of bacteria—we are able to successfully treat many forms of STD's. However, the best "treatment" is the one which requires no treatment—prevention.

Complacency is one of the great fears that I have as a physician. Too many people believe that STD's can be easily treated. They can't. Not always. Many that can be treated do damage to the body before treatment which cannot be reversed. Others cannot be treated successfully.

However, it is easy to say that the best thing to do is abstain from non-monogamous sexual relations. The problem is that our sex drive is too often too powerful—and our monogamous relations are too often unsatisfactory.

Take another of my patient's, Sally, as an example. At fifty years of age, Sally was the last person you would have expected to have gotten herself in a sexual relationship which unraveled her health and her world. But she did.

She was quick to give herself the blame—for everything. When she came to my office, she sat down and even before attempting to speak she was visibly upset.

"It's all my own doing," she repeated several times. "I deserve all the blame. I understand that much..."

Ours was a difficult first interview. She broke down in sobs repeatedly. In between her crying, she managed to weave a story of her life. Her husband, Harry, was an alcoholic. Although he had tried a number of times to get help during their twenty year marriage, he had been unable to find any lasting success.

"He tried them all," she said. "AA. Private counseling. Group counseling. Every quack remedy he found. Nothing did much good.

"Oh, there were times when he would manage to stay sober for weeks, even months, at a time. But then his resolve would be undermined. Something would happen... everything would happen. And he'd be back where he started—only more discouraged.

"Then he'd muster himself to try to find help again. It never lasted," she sighed. "He'd be off on a binge that could last days and days.

"I tried," she told me, imploring me with her tone and her expression to understand just how hard she had tried to help him. "I would scream. I would threaten. I would beg. Plead. Cajole. I would do everything and anything I could think of. But nothing worked. Nothing changed.

"He's in another program now but I have no real hope." She looked at me with the eyes of one who is barely surviving. "I have a twenty-year history of failure. I can't just believe. Not just like that." She drew a deep breath. "I can't imagine ever believing again."

Over the course of their marriage, she was the one who held a steady job. She was the one who was the rock and foundation of their home life. In truth, her job afforded her some sense of sanctuary from her home life.

Working as a librarian in the nearby city college, she was able to interact with young people and be involved with books.

"They were so enthusiastic," she told me. "It gave me hope."

She was especially thrilled when her son, Steve, began attending the college. Their relationship flourished as they established a bond outside the home, a bond that seemed to be built on Steve's future rather than on the rocky past they shared with Harry.

"Everything seemed to be going so well," she said sadly.

Still living at home, Steve would often have his very close friend, Adam, stay over. Adam's mother had died when he was a child and he seemed especially close to Sally.

"Steven. Adam. The young people at the college, they kept me feeling young in spite of the stress of my marriage. They kept me interested in so many things—ideas, music, art..."

It was true that, even as emotional as she was when she

came to me, Sally looked much younger than her years. Her skin had a youthful glow and her eyes, so filled with sadness, looked as if they could easily sparkle with the joy of life.

However, she was burdened with terrible sadness and it showed in the way her shoulders slumped.

"Two months ago," she went on after a long pause, "the boys were at home studying for their final exams. Harry, of course, was off on a binge. We didn't know where he was, when he'd be back... *if* he'd be back. We didn't mention anything, of course. Steven and I shared an unspoken promise not to mention Harry when he was gone.

"I guess it made things easier for both of us.

"In any case, the boys were studying until fairly late. Adam, realizing that they would be studying a while longer for a test he was very worried about, asked if he could spend the night.

"Of course he could, I told him. How many nights had he stayed with us in his life? Hundreds. Sometimes I joked that he was my second son. So, I went to bed and told them not to be up too late studying.

"My bedroom is separated from Steven's by a bathroom. I guess you should have a picture of that much in your mind. Maybe in a different house things would have been different. I don't know.

"I never slept particularly well when Harry was off drinking. As difficult as it was when he was home, I couldn't help but feel a little more secure when he was there. So, I was tossing and turning through another restless night when my bedroom door opened slightly.

"Standing there, dressed only in his underwear, was Adam. I glanced at the clock. It was two in the morning. I asked him if he was all right. He shrugged.

"I could see he was worried. I was sure he was anxious about the exams and how a poor performance would affect his ability to transfer to a good, four-year college. Since I wasn't able to sleep either, I invited him to come down to the kitchen for a glass of warm milk. I thought that might help both of us a little bit.

"I threw on a robe and gave him one of Harry's," she said.

Then the two of them went downstairs to the kitchen. As she warmed the milk, Adam sat down at the table and they began to have some small talk. They talked about Adam's concerns about the test and even a little about how hard it had been growing up in a house without a mother.

Finally, Sally suggested that Adam go back and try and get some rest. "It's going to be a difficult enough day," she said. "You'll need whatever rest you can get."

He nodded. "Thanks. You're the greatest."

When he got up from the table, he went over to hug her. Sally returned the hug, feeling a warm caring for Adam. However, when she began to release her embrace, his arms tightened around her. He leaned toward her and pressed his lips against hers.

She could feel the lump of his erection against her thighs.

"I know I should have pushed him away," Sally told me, hanging her head in shame. "I could have done it without hurting his feelings... but it wasn't his feelings that I was thinking about." She looked at me with an imploring expression on her face. "It had been *two years* since I'd had sex with Harry. Two years.

"Doctor, I'm not a young girl but two years is a long, long time to go without sexual relations. I.. I couldn't seem to help it. My body just reacted to him. My knees trembled. They trembled. And not just with discomfort at the situation.

"I felt such a powerful urgency," she confessed.

Then, with downcast eyes, she explained how she and Adam went to her bed and made love several times before morning.

"I sent him back to Steven's room so that my son wouldn't become suspicious when he woke up and discovered that Adam wasn't there."

Sally didn't know how she managed to make it through preparing and serving the boys breakfast. "I tried to do everything just like I always did but of course *nothing* was like it always was.

"I felt such a deep, deep sense of shame. I didn't know what to say—or do. I mean, I was supposed to be the grown-up. I couldn't help but think what terrible advantage I'd taken of Adam.

"How could I? How could I have sex with a boy, a *boy*, thirty years younger than I am? And my son's best friend!"

She shook her head sadly.

"Of course, Steven didn't suspect a thing. How could he? He even asked if Adam could stay over so they could study together until the exams were over—two weeks later.

"I couldn't say no. That would have given us away. So for the next two weeks Adam slept over and he and I had sex every night. If Harry was on a drinking binge I was on a sex binge. We even continued after Harry staggered home from his own bout.

"We did it everywhere and anywhere we could. In bathrooms. Downstairs in the den. Even in the laundry room on top of the dryer..."

She described Adam as a dream lover, far more sensitive and tender than any man Sally had ever been with.

"I just responded so completely to him." She drew a deep breath. It wasn't long before she had abandoned her sense of shame. Unfortunately, with her sense of shame went caution.

Steven finally discovered them. He came into the kitchen early one morning to find his mother astride Adam on a kitchen chair, her left breast in Adam's mouth.

"If you could have seen the look on his face..." Sally said sadly. "I.. I can't bear to think about it but I can't get it out of my mind either."

Steven just stared for what seemed like hours but then he gave a loud, guttural scream, "No!" and ran from the room. He grabbed his coat and his backpack and ran from the house.

Adam, tucking in his shirt, ran after him.

"Oh, I knew it was over then," Sally said, her voice betraying the depth of the finality she felt. "It was over all right. Everything was over."

She knew that she wouldn't enjoy sex with Adam again. She knew that her relationship with her son would be very damaged. And Harry?

"He was the only one I didn't concern myself with," she said.

Two weeks later, she began to suffer from vaginal itching, burning and soreness on urination as well as signs of discharge in her panties.

"My God, I deserved to have the plague come down on me," she said, crying softly.

I tried to comfort this poor woman. She was clearly suffering from a deep sense of guilt and responsibility over what had happened. And, while it was appropriate for her to take responsibility for her behavior, she needed to put her behavior in perspective.

She had struggled with a horrible marriage for many years. Now, she was struggling with the aftermath of her sexual "binge".

Had she done something "wrong"? I suppose some people would think so but such judgments should not be made without consideration given to her. No individual should be compelled to go without enjoying sexual relations.

Harry's alcoholism was a primary cause for what was unsuccessful in that household.

Even after trying to comfort her, I had to examine Sally and determine what she was suffering from. Although her symptoms might have, on first glance, seemed similar to those of other patients, her lab results indicated that she was suffering from trichomoniasis, a widespread STD that is, at its base, a vaginal infection.

I prescribed the appropriate medication. Six months later, I received a note from her. In it, she thanked me for my kindness and consideration. "Although I may not have expressed it at the time, your understanding was more important to me than the medicine you prescribed to treat my infection."

She wrote that, though it wasn't easy, she and her son managed to talk about what had happened. "He forgave me," she wrote. "He really is a wonderful young man."

She and Harry were attending Al-Anon meetings together. She could only hope that this time Harry could conquer his alcohol demons once and for all.

She did not mention Adam.

10

SYPHILIS

Syphilis is too often the "terrorist" STD. Sometimes referred to as pox, lues, syph, or simply "bad blood", it is far too easily overlooked—often resulting in devastating physical damage.

The disease itself is caused by *reponema pallidum*, a spirochete. True to its terrorist label, the first sign of the disease if usually a single, *painless*, sore called a chancre. Mistaken for a pimple—or not noticed at all—this sign can be the only early chance a patient has to stop any destruction from the disease.

Transmission of syphilis is through intimate contact. Sometimes something as simple as a kiss can be enough for transmission. If you kiss a person who has primary or secondary syphilitic lesions on the lips or in the oral cavity, the disease can be passed along to you.

That's right. Something as simple as a kiss.

A deep, wet kiss is more likely to allow for the transmission of the disease but even a kiss on the lips could be enough given the right circumstances.

Nonsexual transmission of the disease has been documented when a pregnant woman passes the infection to her baby. There have also been cases when the disease is passed along through blood transfusion. However, this is rare due to methods of blood storage.

Under conditions of blood cause storage, the spirochete of syphilis will die within hours. Additionally, modern testing of the blood supply minimizes any risk of contamination.

Sexual transmission is the primary method that syphilis is passed from one person to another.

The easily dismissed chancre sore appears on whatever part of the body where the spirochete has entered. To make it even less likely to be associated with sexual contact, it may appear anywhere from ten to ninety days after contact with an infected person.

In other words, nearly three months after contact, you might see a small chancre sore. Will you make the connection?

How about if the sore disappears by itself, without treatment? Won't you be even more likely to dismiss it as "nothing"?

Unfortunately, while the sore disappears the disease does not. From its primary stage it enters the secondary stage during which a rash or sores may appear on the body. One of the most important diagnostic signs of second stage syphilis is enlarged neighboring lymph nodes, which become hard and tender.

Other symptoms include fever, sore throat, headache, tiredness and temporary loss of hair.

These symptoms can too often be dismissed as flu-like as well, leaving you still vulnerable to the damage of the infection.

This second stage occurs two to six months after sexual contact with the infected person. During the primary and secondary stages, you are extremely infectious to others. However, because the symptoms can appear relatively mild and because they *will disappear* even without treatment, you may not seek medical treatment.

However, *even symptomless, the disease is still present* in your body. Without intervention, you could eventually arrive at stage three syphilis which can result in syphilitic insanity, paralysis, heart disease and even death.

Fortunately for Justina, I was able to treat her syphilis but that didn't make the underlying consequences of her sexual affair any less difficult for her to have to deal with.

At thirty-five, Justina is an attractive woman. A wife and mother, there is much to envy in her life. Unfortunately, the wonderful exterior masked her sense of being neglected by her husband.

As she shared her story with me in my office her overwhelming emotion was deep sadness.

"I made a very bad mistake," she admitted. "A terrible mistake. I'm sure this is God's punishment for that..."

Many times my patients will presume that their STD is an indication of God's punishment for their "wrongful" behavior. As a physician, I do not make moral judgments, only judgments based on medical evidence and my own experience. It is true that a number of my patients come to me because they suffer from diseases contracted in situations they might, in retrospect, have preferred not to be involved in. However, they fail to realize that they were responding to an urge as deep and primal as hunger.

I do not understand how people can think that going without sex for long periods of time is not as difficult as going without food. Ah, but that is what our culture imposes, the sense that the one is to be denied while the other can be sated.

How can people be expected to behave "appropriately"?

The guilt that Justina felt was far out of proportion to her illness. No person should feel neglected as she did. But, let me let her tell her story.

"I had an affair," she said simply. "I don't know why it happened, but it did. And it happened so quickly, so unexpectedly.

"I suppose my situation at home pushed me to it, but still... I shouldn't have... it wasn't right." She raised her sad eyes to me. "What am I going to do now? I know the affair is over...

"I mean, I'm glad... relieved... that it's over but I'm still so upset. About everything. I just don't know what to do. I'm beside myself..."

"Why don't you tell me what happened?" I suggested gently.

"I received a phone call about a week ago from my lover. He said that he had a disease, a sexual disease. I couldn't believe it. I said what's the matter with you? You're a married man... how could you...?

"I could hear the change in his voice when he told me that his wife, like me, was having an affair.

"Well, I didn't believe him at first. I thought he was only trying to get out of our affair. Even that would have been all right, I guess. I don't know. I hated the affair as much as I loved it....

"If only my husband didn't have to work so hard..."

She described her husband as solid and dependable. She swore that she really loved him.

"We always had a good, loving relationship," she said.

He had only just graduated from law school and the long hours he'd put into studying were dwarfed by the hours he had to work to build his practice.

"It was like he was working day and night," she said.

Justina too, had to work. After their children were born, she worked part-time to help make ends meet but also to be able to spend time with her children.

"But even with me working, he didn't slow down a bit. And you know what was worse? He didn't share much about his work with me. It was like we were on parallel tracks. He cared about his work and never shared it with me. And he didn't seem to care much about what was happening with me.

"We never argued. We have never been the kind that fought. I just felt... I just felt that I was being neglected and that he was too busy and too insensitive to my feelings. I didn't feel like he and I were on the same team.

"I mean, I knew why he had to work so much but we had to have *some* time together if we were going to be a family."

Compounding her sense of being neglected and isolated was the fact that she had always relied on her husband for her sexual experience.

"I was a virgin when I met Paul," she said. Even so, the sexual experience with him was not everything that she had dreamed it would be. She had never experienced an orgasm with her husband.

"I never complained about that," Justina said. "I knew that one day it would happen. I just tried to be a perfect, uncomplaining wife." She shrugged. "I tried to turn my energies to the children and to work.

"Work was the real salvation for me. I enjoyed what I was doing and the people there seemed to really care about me. They told me how smart and nice I was. They were quick to compliment me and tell me that I was doing a great job.

"Eventually, I took on more and more responsibility."

With Justina's increased responsibility came travel demands.

"Not long ago, I told Paul that I had to go on a business trip. He was particularly annoyed because he knew that meant he would have to juggle taking care of the kids as well as work.

"He always resented when I had to go away but he especially resented it this time. Maybe because this trip was overseas to England. He told me it was a waste of time for me to go. He said I had a job, not a career and that I shouldn't devote so much time or energy to it.

"He made me feel like I was really nothing to him but his maid and his bed partner.

"When I was in England, I met Corey, a representative from a major corporation. Corey is forty-five, tall and slim. He is every bit a gentleman.

"We spoke briefly and then he invited me to dinner. He brought me flowers and talked to me like an equal, asking me questions about things I cared about.

"After dinner, he asked me up to his hotel. He had this huge, magnificent suite. He ordered champagne from room service and toasted me when it arrived. I guess I should have realized what was going on. After all, there I was drinking in a man's hotel room, a man I'd only known for a day or so. Still, when he kissed me, it took me by surprise.

"At first, I resisted but only half-hearted. It wasn't long before I returned his kisses with passion. As we kissed, he was undressing me.

"You have to remember, sex was not a big deal for me. And, initially, it wasn't that big a deal with Corey. I liked how he was considerate of me and stuff. But then he started doing things to me that my husband *never* did, like kissing me between my legs and stimulating my clitoris.

"I don't know what happened. I felt like I was transported. I was screaming in ecstasy. A wave of passion came over me like I'd never known before. And that's when he inserted his penis into me. I came for the first time in my life. I couldn't even be sure if I didn't actually black out for a moment or two. it was unbelievable. Certainly something I will never forget.

"After that night, I've been with him often. First, we would have lunch before having sex in a nice hotel near the office.

"And you know, my husband didn't even suspect a thing. He was still working very hard. I could have been a ghost for all he knew.

"Well, with my husband a non-presence in my life, I became addicted to Corey. I couldn't seem to get enough... and then he called me with this news.

"Well you can be sure I examined myself closely but I didn't find anything so I thought he'd been making it up. He just wanted out of the relationship. But then my husband complained about a sore on his penis.

"Then I got scared. I told him it was probably from catching himself in the zipper of his pants—and you can bet I was praying that it was. But he was also complaining about swollen glands in his groin.

"About a week later, my husband called me during the day and asked me to meet him during lunch. When I tried to beg off, he said it was an emergency so I said all right.

"'What exactly are all these business trips about?' he demanded. I didn't know what to say. I asked him what he meant and he told me that Kelly, Corey's wife, had called him and told him everything.

"After speaking with her, he'd gone to the doctor and discovered that he had gotten syphilis—from me!

"He was so angry that he picked me up by my hair and hit me—hard. In the face. The bruise is finally beginning to fade."

Justina lowered her eyes. "It's all my fault. What kind of person am I to cause this must pain to people?"

What kind of person indeed. The answer is, simply, a sexually active person. A sexually active person who was, essentially, driven to an illicit relationship because of emotional neglect in her marriage.

Although sex is a physical act, it is not solely a physical experience and most people are as much driven to sexual relationship by emotional needs as by physical needs.

They really cannot be separated. They are continuums of the same thing.

That is the case with almost every patient I see. As I have said, many wish that, in retrospect, they had not become involved in the sexual relationship that caused they to become sick. However, if they hadn't become sick, most of them would never have wanted the relationship to end.

There is a way to do both. But it requires that you be knowledgeable about sexually transmitted diseases and in ways to avoid them.

11

Venereal Warts

One aspect of sexual development that we often react to in damaging ways is the sexual development of young people. Often, in an attempt to blunt the budding sexuality of their children, parents are overly strict. Unfortunately, this type of overbearing behavior can result in consequences no one would have wanted. That was certainly the case with one young woman who came to me not long ago.

Mary is seventeen-years old. She is a good student and is looking forward to college and a wonderful future.

And she is pregnant.

"I don't see why I shouldn't have my baby," she said to me in between gentle sobbing. "I can take care of it."

"But you have your whole future ahead of you—college..."

"Why can't I do both?"

It was a difficult question. Clearly, the statistics would not be in her favor. Few things diminish the future of young women as much as having children before the are intellectually, emotionally or financially ready. Still, there are exceptions.

But those exceptions usually had the support of family. Mary didn't have that. In fact, one might suggest that her family's feeling toward her sexuality contributed to the situation she found herself in.

Enrolled in college prep courses and excelling in sports, particularly tennis, Mary had every reason to look forward to the future. She had a happy childhood. It wasn't until she was older that the strictness of her parents became uncomfortable.

Her mother and father became so strict with her that they checked her menstrual calendar carefully. If she was off by a day or two, her father began a long and uncomfortable inquisition about any possible sexual contact she may have engaged in.

"I didn't even know to think it was weird that my parents watched my cycle that closely," she said. "But when I said something to one of my girlfriends, she looked at me like I was from the middle ages."

She related to me one time when her period was late. "I was under a lot of stress. I was in the middle of an intense tennis competition and I'm sure that had some effect on my cycle.

"But my father wouldn't listen to anything like that. God, it was so embarrassing. He accused me of having sex with my boyfriend and refused to listen to me when I denied it.

"He even confronted my boyfriend. Of course my boyfriend denied it. That was the truth. We *hadn't* had sex. We kissed. That's all. I felt guilty when he touched my breasts.

"My father said we were both liars. He forbade me to ever see my boyfriend again. Then he dragged me to the gynecologist for an examination. Well, the examination proved what we had been telling him. My hymen was intact and I wasn't pregnant.

"Not that my father apologized or anything. And he didn't change his mind about my seeing my boyfriend again. I was so angry with him—and my mother. She didn't say anything in my defense. They both acted like they'd done me a favor, like they saved me from sexual hellfire or something.

"My anger hid some of the embarrassment I felt. The gynecologist tried to be helpful but I just couldn't speak with anyone. I just hated everything about my parents because of that."

Not long after this happened, Mary graduated from high school. In addition to her skill in sports, Mary had become quite proficient in Italian. Wanting to continue to improve her Italian skills and also to study art, she persuaded her parents to let her travel to Italy with a girlfriend.

Together, she and her girlfriend rented a room in a small, private home. They considered themselves very fortunate to have found the room. The young family who owned the house treated them like members of the family, making them feel welcome and comfortable.

Alberto, the owner, was only twenty-seven years old. Although he worked in a factory, he was devoted to art and had a small studio in the attic of the house. His wife was a school teacher who spent her time away from work playing with the couple's two young children.

The two children loved both Mary and her friend. Mary also got along especially well with Alberto, often conversing for hours after dinner in Italian.

"You speak beautiful Italian," Alberto complimented her. "Beautiful Italian for a beautiful young lady."

Mary smiled. She loved the attention Alberto gave her.

One day, when Alberto's wife had taken the children on an outing to visit her parents, Alberto went to Mary's room.

"Where is your roommate?" he asked.

She smiled. "She went into the city. There was a bookstore

she wanted to visit."

"And you?"

Mary shrugged. "I didn't feel like going into the city today."

"Perhaps you would like to see a painting I have done. I think you will like it."

"Sure," she said, smiling.

She followed him up to the attic. When she got there, Alberto showed her a painting he had done of her. "I'm afraid it is not very good," he confessed. "It doesn't capture you as well as I would have liked."

But Mary was swept off her feet by the painting. She thought it was very good. She was pleased at how pretty she looked in it. Because of the nature of her upbringing, she'd never really thought of herself as beautiful but there she was, on the canvas, looking so pretty she almost thought of herself as a different person.

"I.. I look so pretty..." she said shyly.

"Pretty? You are gorgeous!" Alberto replied with real enthusiasm. "Look at you. I didn't come close to capturing your beauty. And your figure... ah, so wonderful...." he sighed. "What I wouldn't give for you to model for me..."

Suddenly, he came up to her and began to kiss her passionately. Although she had kissed her boyfriend many times, there was something much different about Alberto's kisses—an urgency, a certainty—which made her knees weak. Almost without realizing he was doing so, he was undressing her until she was naked in his arms.

He held her at arms length for only a moment, drinking in her beauty and then he laid her down on the couch and began to make love to her.

Although the initial penetration was a bit uncomfortable, Mary quickly began to enjoy the experience. She enjoyed it more because she felt that she truly loved Alberto.

After that first time, she went to his attic whenever the coast was clear, making love to Alberto as often as she could. Although she simply enjoyed the experience the first few times, it wasn't long before she experienced her first orgasm.

Alberto had taken it upon himself to teach her the game of making love. He was a wonderful teacher. When he used his tongue to stimulate her clitoris she trembled and began to moan. She had never experienced a sensation like that before.

Soon, she exploded like a fireball.

When she reluctantly ended her vacation, she missed her period and discovered that she was pregnant.

She wasn't disturbed by this knowledge. She wanted Alberto to come to America and marry her. But he said that he couldn't.

"I love you very much," he confessed. "But I cannot leave my wife and my children."

So, saddened, Mary returned home with her girlfriend. She shared with her parents he condition. Needless to say, they were extremely angry with her.

I spoke with Mary about her determination to keep the baby. She was adamant about not having an abortion.

"But my pregnancy isn't why I've come to you," she said. She then described how, three weeks after returning from Italy, she noticed a small wart on the left side of her vagina. Soon after, ten to fifteen of these warts appeared on the right side of her vagina.

"They hurt," she complained. "And they give off an odor. What am I going to do? Will my baby be all right?"

Like Mary, Dennis was inexperienced sexually. At nineteen, he was very anxious about his lack of social skills. He blamed his acne for his low sense of self-esteem. Also, like Mary, Dennis is a good student. A college sophomore, he is enrolled in a premed program.

"I've always had zits," he said. "Since I was fifteen. But there's getting worse now. I thought they'd be getting better now that I'm almost out of my teens..."

He was very upset about his acne and said more than once that he was sure that was the reason that he hadn't had an easy time getting girlfriends.

"I was a virgin a hell of a lot longer than I ever wanted to be, that's for sure," he said.

He made a point of explaining how much he liked girls, becoming very excited in their presence. "But I feel weird sometimes," he went on. "Like, I'll *feel* really excited but I won't get an erection. One time I was kissing this girl and I was so excited but I didn't get hard. It was really upsetting."

When I asked him if he had trouble maintaining an erection in other circumstances he confessed that he masturbated frequently and that he has wonderful sexual fantasies the whole time.

"But then, when I'm with a real girl... I worry I won't be able to keep it up."

His acne had made him shy and had kept him from any number of experiences which would have reassured him. But, he was a very shy nineteen year old whose anxieties were only going to make his concerns worse.

"I have an older brother, you know. Carl. He's twenty-five. He works as an electrician. One time, I told him about all this. He told me not to worry about a thing, that he was going to take care of everything."

Two days later, his brother called him and invited him to go away for the weekend on a fishing trip to George Washington Lake in upstate New York.

"I told him that that sounded great. I was doing a lot of school work and getting away for a couple of days sounded like the best thing I could think of to do."

When his brother came to pick him up, there were three other people in the car. There was Carl's friend, Sam, in the front seat and, in the back, their girlfriends, Jill and Carmela.

Dennis climbed into the back with the girls. Carmela got his attention in a big way. She was about twenty years old and was very pretty. Her strawberry blonde hair was wavy and fell to her shoulders. She had nice breasts and long legs that seemed not to be able to find a comfortable position the entire drive up. She was moving this way and that, pressing her legs against Dennis'.

Carl and Sam kept talking to the three of them from the front seat. The whole drive up was very pleasant. Between Carmela's leg against his and the conversation, Dennis was as happy as he'd ever been.

Carmela seemed to concentrate on Dennis. At one point, she even said he was nice looking, which made him blush.

When they got to the lake, they all busied themselves unpacking and getting set up. The next day, Carl, Sam and Jill went off shopping, leaving Dennis and Carmela alone.

Feeling awkward, Dennis really didn't know what to say to this beautiful girl that he suddenly found himself alone with. She seemed to enjoy his shyness, flirting with him silently for a while. Then, as the morning grew warmer, she asked if he wanted to go out in the boat.

"Sure," he said.

As he motored the boat, Carmela leaned back on the seat. "The sun feels *so* good. I love days like today." She raised herself up and looked directly at Dennis. "I'm glad I'm sharing it with you."

"I.. I'm glad I'm sharing it too," he stammered.

"Why don't we go out to the middle of the lake and enjoy the deep water?" she asked.

Glad to do anything she wanted, Dennis steered the boat toward the middle of the large lake. In spite of the fact it was a bright, sunny day, there were no other boats around. As they came to the middle of the lake, Dennis cut the engine and they floated along in silence.

"Isn't this gorgeous?" Carmela asked, stretching her arms up and twirling in the bright sunshine.

"Yes," he said, referring both to the day and to her.

Without a word, Carmela pulled her tee shirt up over her head, exposing her breasts. "I'm going to get an all over tan," she smiled at him, giving him a knowing wink.

He felt frozen in place. Carmela seemed perfectly comfortable being half-naked in front of him. He, on the other hand, didn't know what to do. He tried to look away but his eyes continually drifted back to Carmela, topless in the deck chair.

After a minute or two, Carmela lifted herself up and shimmied her shorts down her long legs so that she was completely naked.

"I *love* the sun," she cooed.

Dennis was stunned. He didn't know what to think.

She opened her eyes and looked at him. "Do you think I'm pretty?"

"I..I.. yes..."

She smiled. "Listen, why don't you come over here? Don't you want to play with me? Isn't your cock getting hard yet?"

He froze again. His penis *was* becoming erect.

Carmela stroked her hands up and down her long legs. "Do you like my legs? I would love to wrap them around your face."

Dennis felt his breaths coming in quick succession and his heart pounding in his chest.

"Why don't you take your clothes off and come over here. I'd really like you to suck on my tits and fuck me. Come on, baby. I need you."

Dennis looked at me during the telling of this story. "I couldn't believe how strong my urge could be. I mean, this beautiful girl was just laying there naked as the day she was born and she was talking to me like a truck driver.

"I couldn't have imagined anything like this in my best fantasy. In a second she had me so revved up I was practically frothing at the mouth.

"I threw myself on her like some ravenous dog."

"That's right, baby," she cooed to him. "Take it easy. Slow down. Easy. I'm gonna teach you how to satisfy a woman." Carmela eased him back and pushed down on his shoulders until his face was between her legs. "Use your tongue on me," she said, using her index finger to show him exactly where she wanted his tongue.

In a matter of a few short minutes, she was trembling. Soon after, she began to scream. "Oh God, I'm coming!" she cried out. A moment later, she let her head drop back on the deck chair. "Oh, baby. That was fine," she said.

She took a few deep breaths and then she looked him in the eye. "Okay, baby. Now it's your turn. Stick that virgin cock inside me!"

Dennis pointed his erect penis toward Carmela and she guided it in. He started to pump in and out. She coaxed him on. "That's it, baby. Give it to me harder."

"I.. I did it harder and harder and then I orgasmed with this big load. We were both exhausted so we laid down on the deck, panting in the sun. The two of us, naked as two jaybirds.

"Doc, I felt really *good*. Not just physically. I felt like a real man. I was confident. I wasn't a virgin anymore.

"A while later, we got dressed. When I looked around, I was relieved that there were no other boats around. I could hardly believe my good luck—on all counts. The sex, no boats, the day... it was just too good to be true.

"When we motored back to the dock, the others were there waiting for us. My brother was standing that, impatiently tapping his foot on the dock.

"My brother asked if we had a good time in this lighthearted way. I shrugged and said it was okay. You know, Carmela and I talked and enjoyed the sun.

"The remainder of the weekend was uneventful and then we come home. After we'd dropped the others off, my brother turned to me and asked how Carmela had been. I looked at him like what was he talking about. He told me to get off it. He knew everything.

"When I asked him how he knew, he said he'd decided to boost my ego by asking her to help me out. Then he started to laugh. He said there wasn't a better piece of ass than Carmela anywhere. Then he asked me again if she took good care of me.

"I told him that she was incredible. Then I thanked him for making me a real man. Doc, I can't tell you how great I felt... until about three weeks later. I noticed some warts on the head of my penis. I pretty much ignored them for a while but then they started getting bigger."

When I examined Dennis, approximately one-third of his penis was covered with warts.

Both Dennis and Mary suffered from the same STD—venereal warts. Venereal warts are caused by a virus and generally appear on the sex organ from one to three months following exposure to the virus. Small warts can often be treated with appropriate medication—although while the warts themselves do not pose a risk to a developing fetus, the medication can so it is not prescribed during pregnancy.

Left untreated, the warts can spread or become so large that surgery is necessary for their removal. This was the case for both Mary and Dennis.

Because Mary's warts were exacerbated by her pregnancy, the surgery was especially necessary in her case.

In both cases, I was able to successfully treat the STD. However, both patients had markedly different reactions to their first sexual experiences. While Dennis, despite the pain he suffered, looked back on his sexual "initiation" with great pride, continuing to feel like a "real man" now that he was no longer a virgin, Mary had to deal with her parents and their disapproval of her behavior and her pregnancy.

Although she continued to have loving feelings toward Alberto, her parents were even more strict with her at home. In addition, they pressured her to have an abortion. She remained ambivalent about that decision the last time I spoke with her.

12

WHEN SEX IS DEADLY

While the experience Francis was recounted above, the discussion of HIV and AIDS can not be limited to a single experience. There are those who would suggest that Francis had placed himself at great risk by having unprotected sex with a porn star. It is true that unprotected sex with *any* sexual partner, especially a new sexual partner, is not wise but the attitude that Francis' choice of partner was the real problem is one more example of the greatest danger for sexually transmitted diseases—denial.

The sentiment that it was the "porn star" or that Francis was "reckless" just serves to create the false impression that the rest of us—those who do not have sex with porn stars or act recklessly—are not at risk. That is not completely true.

Denial paralyzes our ability to make appropriate decisions and behave in appropriate ways. It can even be the reason that some people fail to educate themselves in ways that can protect them.

We must not shy away from some central realities:

people—young, old, men, women, straight, gay—are sexually active, and;

the sexual urge drives those same people to adventures that are not always as safe as they should be. As a result, everyone else is at risk.

Alice's situation points to this reality.

At thirty years of age, Alice was married and three months pregnant. She was an attorney who worked in the same law office as her husband, Alex. They had worked together for over two years and been married nearly five years.

"We are the perfect couple," she said to me. "I can't tell you how many of my friends have said how much they envy me." She looked at me with very earnest and intelligent eyes. "And I understand why they're saying it. I'm in love with a wonderful man who loves me. I'm going to have our baby. We're financially secure..."

However, there were dark clouds in this perfectly blue sky. Alice came to me complaining about sores that had developed on genitals, vagina and buttocks.

"I mean, I can't stand the way this pregnancy is playing havoc with my hormones. My skin has been a mess from day one. I've got pimples on my face, doctor. I haven't had a pimple since I was fourteen years old..."

When I asked her how long before she had first noticed the lesions on her sexual organs and buttocks she said about three weeks.

"Well, pregnancy can be very disruptive to the hormonal system and that, in turn can affect your skin," I agreed.

However, in the examination room, in addition to the lesions I discovered a suspicious-looking lymph node. Given her symptoms, my immediate thought was first stage syphilis or herpes genitalis.

"I'm going to draw some blood," I explained. "That may give us a clearer picture of what is going on."

She looked at me nervously. "You don't think the sores are just from the pregnancy? I thought you'd give me a cream or something... Is something wrong?"

"The lymph node is something I'd like to be sure about," I said in a reassuring tone. "We'll know more very soon."

When the blood test came back my suspicion was verified. Alice tested very positive for syphilis. The culture I'd taken of the sores indicated syphilis as well. A culture of the lesion indicated herpes genitalis.

When I explained to her what the blood test showed, she was in absolute shock. "How could something like this happen? I've been married for over five years..."

"Alice, I'm sorry but I'm going to have to ask you some very direct questions and I need you to answer honestly," I said.

She nodded her head and focused her attention on me.

"Have you had an affair?"

"Since my marriage? No, absolutely not," she said emphatically. "I love my husband. I would never, ever have an affair." She leaned forward. "Isn't it possible that I got this in some non-sexual way?"

I shook my head. "I'm sorry. No."

"I don't believe this. I mean, I was certainly sexually active before I was married. Who isn't? And Alex was as well. We've been very honest with one another about that. I mean, I've known Alex for ten years. We haven't been together that whole time but since we've been married..."

Alice struggled through our interview, unable to comprehend the diagnosis that I delivered to her. She was even more troubled when I asked if I could draw blood for an HIV blood test.

Her eyes widened. "What are you suggesting?" she wanted to know.

"Alice," I said gently, "I'm not suggesting anything. But you *are* pregnant and you do have an STD. I think it is only prudent that we be overly cautious."

Unfortunately, in this case, overly cautious meant being right on target. Alice's blood test showed that she was positive for the HIV, the virus which causes AIDS.

What had been only a month or so earlier a perfect life had suddenly evaporated into emotional and physical turmoil. The "perfect" family was in deep trouble. This was a horrible tragedy that she had to come to grips with—as did every other member of her family.

As we continued to speak, her story came out as follows:

She had met her husband about ten years earlier at a girlfriend's party. The party was a wonderful success, filled with young, upwardly mobile young people. People who were either in good colleges, looking forward to studying medicine or law or finance, finishing up at law school or starting their professional careers. Alice found herself in the kitchen having an animated discussion with a handsome man about a movie they'd both seen recently.

As they both discovered, they shared a great many interests and before the evening was over, she and Alex had agreed to see each other informally.

They dated one another but not exclusively.

"We didn't even get intimate then," Alice said. "Warm hugs. Some kisses. That sort of thing. But he was so gentle. He never forced any of that. He's not that kind of person."

They enjoyed movies, boating excursions, hiking trips together. The one thing they both loved was that they were able to speak so freely to one another, sharing their hopes and dreams. And they were both thrilled that those hopes and dreams were so similar—for a large family, to live in Manhattan, to always enjoy theater and museums.

"He was my dream man," Alice said. "And he has been for the entire time I've known him."

Their relationship and their life had been perfect until recently. After Alice's diagnosis, Alex was tested as well. He was positive for all three STD's—syphilis, herpes, and HIV.

Alice looked at Alex. "What's going on?" she asked.

He lowered his head. He raised it two or three times only to lower it again without speaking.

"Do you have girlfriend?" Alice asked in a small, frightened voice.

Alex raised his head quickly. "No. No, I don't have a girlfriend. I.. I.."

Slowly and with great difficulty, Alex confessed that he was bisexual and, while he hadn't been with another woman since they'd been together, he'd been with many men.

Only on a subsequent visit did Alice recall that they sometimes liked to go together to Greenwich Village where Alex would try to coax her into a gay bar.

"I'd always resist. I couldn't see the attraction. I mean, it was all so strange to me. When I asked him why he wanted us to go in, he would joke and say he just wanted to see those faggots. He called them faggots."

She began to cry.

"I guess he was trying to tell me then, wasn't he? He was trying to share something with me that he couldn't bring himself to say out loud. Oh God, what's going to happen to us?"

Only after these terrible diagnoses was Alex able to finally confess that he often went to gay bars and pornography houses where he had anonymous homosexual contacts with a large number of men.

He said that he'd known he was gay when he was thirteen years old but he'd worked hard to hide his nature. "The closet was the perfect place for me. Or so I thought," he said ruefully.

It was his desire to keep his true sexual nature secret that led him to convince himself that he was bisexual. Loving Alice —which he truly did—gave him the perfect "cover". Marriage.

Alice revealed to me that there were other clues about his sexual orientation that were more obvious only now, in retrospect. "We didn't have sex very often and when we did it wasn't very passionate. Alex was more passionate about the last movie we'd seen than physical contact with me.

"I was the one who had to initiate sexual intimacy. And even then we'd only have sex every few months. I didn't worry about it too much. After all, we worked so hard..."

She shook her head. "When we did have sex, he left the bed immediately after and went into the bathroom to wash himself. I guess I should have understood that he found sex with me revolting. I guess I just couldn't accept that..." She began to cry.

Alice and Alex spoke openly—if painfully—about the juncture they had reached in their lives. Although he was now convinced that his desire to be bisexual was hopeless, that he was a gay man, he did have a deep emotional attachment to her.

"I genuinely believed that we could always be together and have the family we both dreamed of," he told her. "I think I was always hoping that I wouldn't be gay anymore, that somehow I would change."

I treated both Alice and her husband for syphilis but the disease had many complications because it was co-existing with the HIV virus. Their herpes genitalis became systemic herpes.

Alex had to be hospitalized so he could receive intravenous antiviral medication.

The aggressive treatment worked—they symptoms of syphilis and herpes were eradicated. Their baby was delivered by cesarean section. A son.

Unfortunately, our success against the syphilis and herpes could not be duplicated against HIV. In about a year and a half, they both developed AIDS. Their complications from the disease included pneumonia, weight loss and candidiasis.

Less than two years after that initial diagnosis, both Alex and the baby had died.

Alice was never in denial. She was committed to a monogamous relationship with the man she loved. However, she never knew her husband's true sexual nature. And, he was unable to share it with her.

In this case, ignorance was both cruel and final.

13

A Doctor's Role in the Treatment of STDs

While my training like the training every M.D. receives—is in the healing of the body, my particular field of medicine brings me into the most intimate details of my patients' lives. As you can see from some of the experiences of my patients, they are often physically and emotionally painful, wrenching to themselves and their partners and family and more than once resulted in the most horrible indignity—death.

While it is true that knowledge could save many of my patients from the ravages of disease, it is also true that they are driven by powerfully human passions. These passions are certainly tied in with libido, with sexual desire. But they are also expressions of profound needs—the need for self identification, the need to find expression for that sense of self, the need to not be lonely.

John, the patient who was in a "happy marriage" with a wonderful woman still felt compelled to be a transvestite and to engage in homosexual behavior. Neither of these decisions were conscious. They were the result of powerful psychological—even genetic—impulses. For this reason, no one should place themselves as judge over John or any other patient or person.

While the specifics of John's experience might be different than another persons, there are few people who have not fantasized of things they would be ashamed to describe in public, few people who have not had a close relationship with another person which did not blur the lines between friends and lovers.

How many women have lingered over the sight of a friend in a changing room or in a swimming pool? Doing so does not suggest that either of the women would be classified as lesbian, just that the spectrum of *normal* human sexuality and desire is much broader than most people would like to admit.

As a doctor who treats patients who have come to suffer for their sexual behavior, I *never* judge. I do, however, often find myself in a role for which I did not receive formal training—that of human counselor. Often, my patients will speak to me about the confusions and fears that are part and parcel of their behavior.

You remember Chloe. Her story when she came to me was that she had gotten very, very drunk and her boyfriend told her that her dog had had sexual relations with her. Above and beyond her what turned out to be her promiscuity, Chloe clearly partied much too much.

More even than this, I found it very interesting that, upon her telling the story to me, she did not seem to have any particular revulsion to having engaged in a sex act with a dog. Of course, this was a particularly significant clue that suggested that the story itself was false—as it turned out to be.

Chloe had had a rendezvous with another man and had

sought to cover it up with a wild story which involved her dog.

As much as I served as doctor, because of the nature of the disease I was treating, I also became something of a "confessor".

After all, the diseases my patients have contracted do not come from "dirty toilet seats." They come from sexual activity. Sometimes the sexual activity is the result of perfectly "normal" and acceptable sexual relations—as between Sarah and Michael. Other times there are adulterous relations involved. Multiple partners. Homosexual experiences.

Are any of these "wrong"?

In the mind of the red-haired preacher, almost all of them are wrong. But in my mind, none of them can be considered wrong. They are activities pursued in the hope of experiencing pleasure, in the desire to ease loneliness or unhappiness, in the search for exhilarating experiences.

Sex is a wonderful thing. It is not an experience limited to people with perfect bodies—thin women with perfectly-shaped breasts and smooth thighs or men with "monster" genitalia. It is an experience that is enjoyed—relished, in fact—by every mammal on earth. None more so than we humans.

My patients range from petite to obese. They come in all colors, from every social, ethnic and demographic background. They are men, women and individuals who choose to blur the line between the two. Men come to me with sores on their penises, some of which are enormous while others are much more modest.

All our culture's definition of beauty manages to do is to inhibit people who do not fall within that narrowly defined notion of beauty or sexiness. That, along with some very repressive messages delivered when he was a young boy, conspired to keep Francis a virgin until he was willing to do just about anything in order *not* to remain a virgin, including engage in behavior without any thought to his physical well-being.

We live at such an awkward time. I have spoken to the strange notion of "perversion" as highlighted in recent national events. People shy away from healthy sexual appetites because they are convinced they are not pretty or that they are not sexy or that what their imagination tells them they want they are convinced is wrong.

What is wrong is that people should suffer needlessly for pursuing their desires.

The intensity of an orgasm. The pleasure of physical contact. The emotional release of sex. These are all realities of the sexual act—not of the way those engaged in the physical act *look*.

My perspective regarding sexual activity is very simple—while I recognize that some sexual activity carries with it real physical risks, I do not *ever* view consensual adult sexual activity as a moral issue. Therefore, when my patients come to me, I counsel them regarding how their decisions might affect their health. I never judge them.

What I hope to do—in addition to healing their bodies—is to educate them.

There was a time when we believed that we would gain a medical victory over sexually transmitted diseases. Unfortunately, the AIDS epidemic and the appearance of drug-resistant strains of STDs has rendered this belief premature. Victory over disease is the goal in every field of medicine. What we have come to learn is that such victories are few and far between.

Diseases are pernicious and determined. Eradication is not

always possible. Cure is not always available.

In the absence of cures and curative treatments, the best hope is a sound strategy for *avoiding* disease and of preventing its spread. Cures *will* be found but those cures will likely not be available until well into the next century. In the meantime, we must continue to study the nature of STDs, their causes and the best way to prevent their spread.

While the religious moralists would like us to view STDs as the curse of God, they are, simply, like other diseases in that they are caused by organisms (germs). The difference between an STD and another disease has to do with the method of transmission. In other words, how one "catches" it. STDs are transmitted during sexual activity by those who are already infected with such a disease to those who are not.

Traditionally, diseases such as syphilis and gonorrhea were called "venereal diseases."—venereal after "Venus", the goddess of love, by the Victorians who were notably squeamish at the mere mention of "sex" or "sexuality". With the discovery of penicillin—the first effective treatment for syphilis, there arose what we now know only too well to be the erroneous belief that STDs would always be easily treatable with antibiotics, rendering them more like annoyances than real health threats.

Unfortunately, time and experience have brought home the error of that view. None of us can afford the luxury of ignorance when confronted by the threats posed by such sexually transmitted diseases as AIDS and herpes. Indeed, our single most potent weapon to counter the steady rise of these diseases is knowledge.

Several factors have conspired to foster an environment in which the number of STDs could increase. As families and society in general become less structured, the traditional restraints on sexual activity diminish. We are bombarded with an ethos that demands instant gratification, demands that play into the uncertainties of adolescence—a time of physical, physiological, and psychological change. Ignorance about sexual health and disease is coupled with the availability of new forms of contraception, forms which have essentially eliminated the *fear* of unwanted pregnancy (and its subsequent inhibition of sexual activity), though not the *reality* of it.

While the fundamental changes that are occurring in society are extremely difficult to address, we can and must certainly address the issue of ignorance when it comes to sexual health and STDs. To begin, we must address some misconceptions. These diseases exist at *all levels of society*, from the stars of entertainment and industry to the poor and indigent. STDs are not a poor man's disease. Infections cross all lines of age, education, income level, and ethnicity. The danger of contracting these diseases comes not from dirty toilet seats or casual contact but from *intimate, sexual contact*. Indeed, the single greatest risk factor in contracting STDs is having multiple sexual partners. STDs can be transmitted in the absence of traditional, genital-genital sexual intercourse. STDs can be contracted "the first time". STDs can result in impairment of sexual organs, sometimes resulting in sterility or even death. Finally, although we have begun to hear and learn more and more about AIDS many other STDs continue to plague us.

Before STDs can be eradicated, ignorance regarding them must be eradicated. Ultimately, knowledge about STDs must also be a call to action—regarding personal sexual activity as well as public health policy.

Ultimately, we are each foot soldiers in the fight against these diseases. My role is to treat those who have been wounded in this battle—often psychologically as well as physically.

Sometimes that is more difficult than other times.

14

WHEN SEX IS NOT LIFE-AFFIRMING

I had just returned from a lovely stroll in the park. After carefully washing my hands, I stepped into my inner office. When I left for lunch, I believed I would have until nearly 1:30 before I would be seeing my next patient. I was looking forward to the opportunity to catch up on some reading and to finish up some paperwork.

However, my leisurely lunch break was not destined to be. I had no sooner settled at my desk than my nurse stepped into my office.

"Yes?"

"I'm sorry to bother you," she apologized.

"No, no," I assured her, putting down my paperwork, "no bother at all. What is it?"

She glanced back toward the waiting area. "A young woman has come in," she began. "She doesn't have an appointment..."

"So? Why not have her make an appointment and I will be glad to see her," I said.

"She began to explain to Joyce..." she said. Joyce is one of my receptionists. "...she began to explain to Joyce how she thinks she might have gotten sick..."

I looked at her curiously. She, like I, had heard many, many stories and she had never before exhibited anything close to what seemed to me to be a sort of squeamishness and discomfort. "Are you all right?" I asked her.

She clasped her hands together and wrung them anxiously. "I think you should speak with her," she said.

I raised my eyebrows. "Well then, you've gotten me intrigued. Okay, let's get a history and bring her in," I said.

"Thank you," she said.

A short time later, Joyce was showing a very attractive blonde into my office. The young woman appeared a bit sallow and moved slowly, as if she were very tired. I indicated that she should have a seat. She smiled at me as Joyce handed me the brief history that she had filled out. I looked at it briefly and then at the young woman.

"Well, Gwen, how can I help you today?" I asked.

In spite of her good looks, Gwen looked very nervous and uncomfortable. "I.. I don't know where to begin..."

I smiled and tried to put her at ease. "Please," I prompted her. "I can't very well help you if you don't help me," I said.

She looked down at her hands as they rested in her lap. "I.. I've been experiencing increased vaginal discharge," she said.

I nodded. "Okay. That's not an uncommon discomfort."

"I also have an itching inside my vagina and a soreness around my vulva." She glanced up at me almost apologetically. "And I know I look awful. My color's all messed up. I'm tired a lot..." A very worried look came over her. "Am I going to be all right?"

"I certainly hope so," I said reassuringly. "However, the

first thing we're going to have to do is find out what all these symptoms add up to. Is there anything else you can tell me about them?"

"About three weeks ago, I began experiencing a frothy discharge after sex."

"You're sexually active then?"

She nodded.

"Are you in a monogamous relationship?"

She paused for a moment. "Yes and no."

I looked at her curiously. "Yes and no? Does that mean your partner is not monogamous?"

She shook her head. "Oh no. I'm sure my boyfriend isn't screwing around. He wouldn't ever do that to me."

"Is he experiencing any symptoms?"

"His color is sallow like mine," she said.

"And he's monogamous, you're sure?"

"Yes."

I brought my hands together and rested my chin on them. I looked directly at her. "I'm a bit confused then. If your boyfriend is monogamous then..."

She drew a deep breath. She looked directly at me. She began to speak, paused and then started up again. The story she unfolded was one I had never before encountered—and I'd encountered many, many stories.

"I became sexually active my first year in High School," she began. "I was on the cheerleading squad and I started going out with one of the varsity football players. At first, we just fooled around. You know, making out and stuff.

"I didn't really think of sex as something to do itself. It was all part of the whole picture, you know. Football season. The excitement of winning. A cute boyfriend on the team. It wasn't about sex. It was about being popular and all that.

"Anyway, we had sex the first time after the team lost the championship game. My boyfriend was kinda depressed and he was drinking a lot with the whole team.

"He'd been pushing harder and harder for us to go all the way for a while but I'd been resisting... it wasn't that I didn't want to or anything. I guess I just thought, when it came right down to it.. that there was something not right about it." She rolled her eyes. "Well, I was about to change my mind.

"We were at a post-game party and my boyfriend got real drunk. I wasn't drunk but I had some to drink which I'd never done before. Anyway, one thing led to another and we ended up in the back of his friend's van naked under a blanket.

"That was my first time. Pretty romantic, huh?" There was a moment of silence as she struggled with continuing. "After he was finished, he kind of fell asleep. Passed out is more like it.

"I started playing with him... with his penis.. and he got an erection again. But he didn't wake up. I thought that was kind of cool. I ended up having sex with him and he didn't even know it.

"When I told him the next day, he didn't believe me but it was the truth.

"I don't know what happened to him. He went off to college while I still had three years of high school to go. But, I was a pretty cheerleader so I never suffered for attention.

"I had my pick and choose of boys. Plus, the guys knew that I wasn't a virgin so even if I didn't go all the way with them, they knew that we'd do some serious fooling around. Of course, that made all the girls I knew jealous.

"It wasn't like I was a slut or anything. I mean, I didn't just do stuff with guys. We always went out for a while first. Boyfriend-girlfriend. Still...

"I like beautiful men," she blurted out. "It's that simple. I was spoiled young. I like beautiful, athletic, strong guys. I always have." She shrugged. "I guess I always will.

"I've had a lot of sexual relationships over the years but I'm pretty monogamous now. I came east about six months ago to be near by boyfriend. He's a bartender at the Golden Splash Club in Harrison."

"He works as a bartender? Isn't that an environment that could invite someone to be sexually active?"

"Eric's cool," she said with absolute confidence. "We met when we were both on vacation in the Islands. He has this amazing body. I couldn't take my eyes off him from the moment I first saw him by the pool.

"He was wearing these little Speedos..." she smiled. "The first time we made love was on the beach just after sunset. Now *that* was romantic. We were together the entire vacation. After we came back, he visited me in California and I came here to visit him.

"I decided that I was happier near him than away from him so I picked up and came east.

"I had the kind of job that made it easy to relocate."

"What do you do?"

"I'm a pathologist assistant," she said. "I assist in performing autopsies." She shrugged. "There's never an employment shortage in my field. Not in the cities. I interviewed and got a job here on my last visit. Two weeks later, I moved all my stuff and here I was."

There was an incongruity to this pretty, blonde hair California girl working long hours in a cold morgue.

Something about it troubled me but I couldn't quite put my finger on it.

"What got you involved in that field?" I asked.

"Two things," she said. "I was pretty good with make-up and during my senior year in high school, I got a job doing faces at a local mortuary. That kind of got me fascinated with dead people.

"In college, I started pre-med but there was no way I was going to make it to medical school. My grades were all right but they weren't the kinds of grades that would get me in. So, I kind of gravitated to one of the related fields." She laughed. "I couldn't see myself as a dentist!"

Then she lowered her head. "Actually, what it comes down to is I'm a morgue rat, doctor."

"A what?" I asked, not certain I heard her correctly.

"A morgue rat. I'm in love with dead people. I'm fascinated by them. I'm attracted to them." She brought her hands together. "I have sex with dead men," she said softly. Then she raised her eyes to mine. "Is that so weird? I'm in love with beautiful, dead bodies."

I didn't say anything. I just waited while she drew in another breath and, after a moment, continued. "There was this one man—hardly more than a boy, actually. He was nineteen years old. He'd been killed in a car accident. Severed spine. But his face was so gorgeous. He hadn't suffered any head trauma and laying on the gurney, he looked like he was sleeping." She giggled nervously. "Maybe his color wasn't so great but no one's color is great under those lights. He really did look like he was sleeping.

"When I lowered the blanket, I could see that he'd suffered trauma to his chest. But when I continued to lower the blanket

I discovered the largest penis I'd ever seen. It was.. it was massive."

"I *have* been to counseling," she said. "But it doesn't change anything. I'm a necrophile. I don't know why. Maybe it was making love in high school with my unconscious boyfriend. My shrink thought it had more to do with when I saw my uncle have sex with my dead aunt.

"God, I couldn't have been more than eleven or twelve. My aunt and uncle had been married for about twenty-five years. She died in a freak accident. The wake was in their house down the block from where I lived.

"After we all left, I went back because my uncle looked so sad. I walked in through the back door and I heard strange sounds coming from the room where my aunt was.

"I snuck up real quiet and I peeked through the key hole. My uncle had pushed up my aunt's dress so she was naked from the waist down and he unbuckled his belt.

"He let his pants fall down to and then he took his penis in his hand. He played with himself for a minute until he had an erection and then he had sex with my dead aunt. I was too excited by what I'd seen to think it was strange or wrong. In fact, when I went home I masturbated for the first time.

"When I was eighteen and a freshman in college, I did volunteer work at the local hospital. I thought it would help when I applied for medical school. Anyway, there was this one day when I was working in the morgue. No one was around and a body had just been brought down.

"This man was so beautiful. And so peaceful. He'd died from a heart attack in his sleep. His whole body was perfect. Not a mark on it. And his penis... " she shook her head slowly as if to indicate that even now she remembered it vividly.

"I started trembling with excitement. I could feel myself getting so wet I didn't know what to do with myself. I considered going into the bathroom to masturbate but here was this man with this beautiful penis just laying there on the table... I made sure that no one was around and then I closed the door. I kept my skirt on but I slipped off my panties. Then I climbed onto the table with him. I straddled him and took his big penis in my hands and managed to shove it into my vagina.

"I moved up and down for several minutes and then had an orgasm. When I was done, I climbed down from the table. I put the blanket over him and I went into the bathroom where I masturbated to another orgasm before cleaning up and putting my panties back on.

"That was the first time I did it with a corpse," she conceded. "But it wasn't my last.

"Since then, I've had sex with several dead men. They are always beautiful and they always have big penises. I had one boyfriend that I shared my sexual habit with. I would have sex with him *and* a corpse. That was pretty wild. Sex with my boyfriend alone was nothing compared to sex with him and a corpse.

Even now, I still have sex with my boyfriend but sex with dead men excites me so much more.

"A few years ago, I had sex with a dead bodybuilder who'd been killed by a stray bullet. I really enjoyed him a lot. The family didn't claim his body for a while so I made love to him several times. I even called him my *dear lover* until he was buried.

"Doctor, I never cheat on my boyfriend with other guys and I know that he never cheats on me. But now I have these symptoms... Could I have caught something from one of my dead lovers?"

I wasn't sure how to answer her. While it was doubtful that she could have contracted a disease from a corpse—as body fluids were not likely to have been exchanged—I could not say conclusively that it was impossible.

"What I'd like to do is to find out exactly what's going on in your body now so that I can treat it and then we can explore the answer to your question," I told her.

A pelvic examination showed that she was suffering from vaginitis—a readily treatable condition.

"I'd like to do a blood work-up and have you come in for a follow-up next week," I told her.

"Thank you," she said. Then she looked at me. "And thank you for listening. I.. I really having been feeling well for quite a while but I couldn't bring myself to go to a doctor... I was scared how he'd react."

I gave her case a great deal of thought—both ethically and medically. Ethically, I did not believe what she did was right. Without engaging in any discussion of right or wrong, good or bad, her behavior involved people who had not consented to engage in it. The fact that they were deceased only made them more vulnerable and therefore more deserving of protection.

Medically, her situation posed an interesting question. Could she contract an STD from a corpse? Her blood work made the question much more of an issue. I had to inform her that she had advanced hepatitis and also suffered from HIV.

Although no body fluids were exchanged with the corpse, certainly no semen was ejaculated from the corpse. However, there existed the very real possibility that blisters or pockets of fluid still remained on the corpse's penis. Certain viruses, like the HIV virus, are very fragile and cannot live for very long in anything but near-perfect conditions. Other viruses however, like hepatitis, can live for as long as two weeks outside the human body.

Clearly, there was the possibility that certain diseases could be transmitted—albeit passively—from a corpse to Gwen. In addition, the probability of such an exchange depended in part with how long the person had been dead before she had sex with him.

More than once, Gwen had engaged in a sexual act with a corpse just brought down to the morgue. In these cases it was possible that an active virus was transferred to her.

Of course, one needed to remember that Gwen was still fairly promiscuous and had been for most of her young adult life. Although she tended to be monogamous with her current (living) boyfriend, she had engaged in sexual activity with many men over her life. Any of them could have been the source of the diseases she was suffering from.

Although Gwen still looked very pretty when I first met her—like a beautiful girl getting over a bout of the flu—she was much sicker than her appearance indicated. Four months after I first spoke with her, she died. The primary cause of death was liver failure brought about by the hepatitis.

I am the kind of doctor who cares deeply about his patients. Although I, like most doctors, see a large number of people over the course of a day and a week, I believe I get to know each of my patients as an individual. Doing so is a challenge for all doctors, myself included. However, it is made easier for me because of the nature of my interaction with patients. They share with me such intimate aspects of their lives it would be impossible for me *not* to get to know them as individuals.

I remained haunted by Gwen for a long, long time. Not only with the sad fact that she died from a disease which might have been treatable but because I constantly struggled with the ethical aspect of her behavior.

Sexuality is threatening to people because it exists at the nexus of powerful aspects of who and what we are. Sexual behavior must, therefore, sometimes challenge what the culture states as being normal. Even though I have yet to meet a person who has a "normal" sexual relationship or possess "normal" sexuality we have a cultural investment in having some faith in the existence of such a norm.

As a doctor who treats sexually transmitted diseases in people who have stepped outside that "norm", I respect their needs, desires, drives and emotions on face value. As I've said over and over, I do not judge my patients. Or people who are not my patients for that matter.

Yet I remain troubled by Gwen. I cannot condone any behavior—sexual or otherwise—which trespasses on the rights of others. I am a champion of the rights of any adult to engage in any consensual sexual activity. But Gwen took advantage of individuals who could not consent. It is true that neither could they protest but in either case, I believe she committed a trespass.

I do not believe that it was her necrophilia which resulted in her death. I believe that the STDs that she'd contracted were most likely contracted by a living lover.

The epidimiological issue she raised was an interesting one. And the most interesting aspect of it? That it had a very real human face. Hers.

It is the humanity of these things which make them compelling. And I cannot erase Gwen's face from my mind.

15

WHEN A HARMLESS FETISH CAN BE DANGEROUS

People become fascinated by many things. I once met a man who had become an expert at ornamental hood decorations on classic cars. Another on the various gargoyles that protect European churches. Their growing fascination caused them to become ever more specific about the tiniest aspect of these things. A man I had known in school became a professor of literature. His area of expertise was in the use of verb structures in Romantic Poetry.

When I questioned this man who had devoted so much time and energy to what could only be viewed as an almost trivial thing to the non-initiate, he smiled and said, "My friend, God is in the details."

It is true. When we are fascinated by a thing, our fascination often drives us to greater and greater specificity. Few men are attracted to all women. They find greater beauty in blondes or in women with large breasts or in women with small breasts, women with long legs and shapely behinds or overweight women with double chins. There is a popular television series on television now in which a character is powerfully moved by the particular shape and texture of the skin under a woman's chin.

Woman are attracted to men who earn a great deal of money, who have powerful chests, who hold important positions, who have large penises. Other women are most attracted to the shape of a man's lips or his eyes and say "size does not matter to me."

In other words, there are multitudes of specific areas of attraction, of focus. When a particular *object* because the source of incredible fascination and attraction, we call it a fetish.

For the most part, fetishes are harmless. A woman has a large collection of shoes, which she has acquired because of the sensual pleasure she derives from shoe stores and trying shoes on. A man has a shoe fetish, getting sexually excited by the touch, feel, smell of a woman's shoes. He might get an erection and actually use a shoe to masturbate.

Anything can be the object of a fetish. One very common object for men is women's underwear. Specifically panties. That was the case for a patient who came to me not long ago.

Nathan, at fifty years old, was hardly the picture of who the average person would expect to come to a doctor with a concern about sexually transmitted diseases. Not only was Nathan a bit past his prime, he was balding and overweight. During his best years he would never have been cast as a sexually dominant individual. At five foot four, with a soft voice that still bore the traces of a childhood lisp, Nathan seemed to be exactly what he was—a very considerate accountant.

Never married, Nathan's sexual experiences were few and far between. He did, however, have an active sex life, one that depended on masturbation and his fascination with women's panties.

"I guess I knew early on that I was a fetishist," Nathan told me. "When I was a kid... heck, thirteen or fourteen, I used to take my mom's underwear out of the hamper and masturbate with it." He colored slightly. "You don't think I'm a pervert, do you?"

I shook my head. "No, not at all."

He seemed relieved. "Well, you're in the minority, I'll tell you that. I went to a shrink for a long time. *He* thought I was a pervert all right. By the time he was finished with me I felt guiltier than I had when I started with him.

"I can't help it," he said emphatically. "I get so damned aroused by women's underwear. I send away for all those things advertised in the back of magazines—you know, the ones where they'll send you used underwear... I like seeing women in their underwear too but that's not nearly the turn on of the underwear alone.

"One time, I was working late in the office. No one else was there. I was walking past the ladies' room as I was headed to the men's room when I happened to stop and open the door. I don't know why just something made me do that.

"I didn't go in right away. I looked around. God, I don't know what I would have done if I'd been caught. I'd have been so mortified... I mean, the janitorial staff was in the building somewhere. At least, I assumed they were. But I hadn't seen anyone for a while and there didn't seem to be anyone around right then so I went inside.

"It was gleaming clean. Nothing particularly noteworthy. I assumed that the janitors had already been in to clean but then I saw something that almost caused my heart to stop. In one of the stalls, on the floor, I caught a glimpse of something. I went closer. Carefully, I pushed open the door of the stall. There on the tile floor near the back of the toilet was a pair of panties.

"God, I almost passed out! They were an off-white color. Cotton, with lace around the leg openings. They were bikini type. I grabbed them and brought them to my nose. I could *smell* the scent of a woman on them. The crotch was still moist. There was a very pale stain in them—one that had been nearly washed out long ago.

"You can't imagine how I felt. I was immediately aroused. My erection was pushing so hard against the zipper of my trousers that it hurt.

"I didn't give any thought to where I was or the danger—I undid my belt and let my pants fall to the tops of my shoes. I began to masturbate with one hand while I held the panties against my face with the other.

"When I was about to orgasm, I wrapped the panties around my penis and stroked myself until I orgasmed into the cotton. I was so weak in the knees it was several moments before I began to think straight again. When I did I realized the danger I had put myself in.

"I quickly pulled up my trousers and tucked my penis in. I straightened myself up and stuffed the panties into my coat pocket. After making sure the coast was clear, I hurried from the ladies room back to my desk. I quickly put the panties in my briefcase. Then I went back to the men's room to relieve myself.

"The remainder of the time I worked that evening I was in a semi-aroused state because of those panties. I kept thinking about them in my briefcase. I wondered who they had belonged to—I narrowed it down a little because of their size.

I was just beside myself trying to think of how and why whoever had been wearing them had taken them off and left them in the bathroom.

"Was she maturbating at work? The thought of it had me rushing back to the men's room to masturbate again.

"For weeks afterward, I watched the eyes of all the women in the office, trying to catch their eyes to see if I could elicit a response to find out if who had left the panties there. That turned into a real game for me, one that took up countless hours of office and home time.

"It gave me shivers trying to figure out which woman would wear that kind of panty. It was all so marvelously intriguing."

"What would you have done if you'd discovered who the panties had belonged to?" I asked him.

He colored slightly. "Oh goodness, I don't know. Probably nothing. I mean, in my fantasies I would have loved to have engaged in mutual masturbation or something like that. Maybe she could have given me other pairs. In my fantasies I imagined that she'd purposefully left her panties there for me. Could you imagine?

"But no, I don't often have relations with women. When I dated my first girlfriend, I was young and very inexperienced. We were at Lisa's apartment, kissing and engaging in heavy petting when she took off her dress. I was breathless. There she was in this beautiful underwear. Matching bra and panties—not that I paid much attention to the bra. Panties are my fascination. The elastic on one of the leg openings had slid over so that her pubic hair, along with the outer lip of her vagina, was visible.

"My penis practically exploded into the firmest erection

you could imagine. It was just throbbing. In spite of her protests, I quickly pulled down my zipper and took out my erect penis. Before I knew what was happening, I came all over her underwear.

"She was very angry—by my behavior and the mess I made on her underwear. That was the end of our relationship but the real maturation of my destructive life style.

"While I was in accounting school, I worked part-time in department stores. At work, I became a peeping Tom, looking through the keyholes in the dressing rooms to see women undressing. It didn't matter if they were young or old, tall or short, fat or thin. Just the idea of them undressing and being in their underwear was enough to get me wildly excited.

"More than once I came in my pants when I saw women in their underwear. I was always so thrilled and guilty at the same time. But I reasoned that my behavior didn't harm anyone so it was all right.

"I even took women's underwear home with me. That seemed sick to me but I did it just the same. I couldn't help it.

"I have more than three hundred pairs in my apartment. Can you believe that? Three hundred pairs! I use them when I masturbate. Most of the time, I only need one pair to get me off—and no women. Panties and my imagination are more than enough to arouse me and make my masturbation wonderful.

"Although I have never been much of a Casanova, I have slept with a few women in my life. Their underwear *really* excited me. I could smell their panties, touch them. I took them off them, rolling them over asses and legs, smelling them the whole time.

"I could take five minutes just sliding a woman's panties

off her, sniffing and licking her—and them—the whole time. Ah, the sweetest sensation in the world! I love women's pussies! I do. But I love them most when they are pressed against the tight material of women's panties.

"I've had women tell me I'm a wonderful lover because of my patience, because of the way I linger over their bodies. They don't understand that I really love their underwear.

"I went out with one women who did appreciate my fetish. After she became aroused, she would rub herself through her panties, making sure that they were damp and thick with her scent. Then she would let me take them off—sometimes commanding me to take them off with my teeth!

"Usually, she let me keep the panties. After a little while she complained that she couldn't afford to keep buying new panties to wear so I used to buy her panties.

"She liked domination games which weren't my favorite turn-on. After a time, we drifted apart and I was left with some wonderful memories—and over a dozen pairs of her panties."

"Of course," he said, "none of this is exactly why I've come to see you today. I.. I have some strange sores all over my penis."

"Why don't we go into the examination room and see," I suggested.

Inside the examination room, Nathan stripped to his boxer shorts while I washed my hands. Then I put on examination gloves and asked him to please lower his shorts.

His penis was covered with multiple warts, fiery red and white with irregular borders. The rash of warts extended to his legs. These warts exuded an order and caused him considerable discomfort, primarily the result of chafing when he walked.

"Please turn around," I asked him.

When he did, I could see that the warts extended around to his anus.

"Other than the warts, do you have any symptoms?" I asked him.

He shrugged his shoulders. "No. None that I'm aware of."

My examination revealed that his lymph nodes were normal and that he had no discharge from his penis.

"When did you begin to experience these symptoms?"

Pulling up his boxers, Nathan sat back down on the examination table. "About three weeks ago, I met a woman. Actually, I met her underwear." He looked at me as if I might not appreciate the significance of the distinction. "I had gone to a topless bar in a neighborhood not far from my home. She was dancing on a small stage. Doc, she was incredible. Practically naked, she was only wearing this tiny pair of thong panties, black with lace...

"I had been about to leave when she started to dance. As soon as I saw her, I couldn't move. My penis started to throb. She was *this close* to me," he said, indicating that she'd been dancing within a few feet of him. God, when she gyrated her pelvis and thrust her panties toward me I though I'd die of pleasure.

"I think I was actually groaning—although the music was so loud no one—including myself—could have heard. Finally I just had to get up and get to the bathroom to masturbate. I had to.

"When I came out, she was finishing her shoe. Doc, I couldn't take my eyes off her—or her panties. I followed her home," he went on, hanging his head. "For the next few days I trailed after. I guess I was almost stalking her," he added sheepishly.

"I saw where she lived, where she ate.

"Finally, in a bar in SoHo, I went up to her and introduced myself. I explained that I'd seen her dance in the bar and that I had been so enamored of her... She seemed to know what I was about immediately. She let me buy her drinks and soon we were both fairly drunk.

"Then she asked me if I wanted to go to her place. I couldn't believe it. Of course I said yes. I would have walked through fire at that point.

"Once we were in her apartment, she asked me what it was that I liked most about her dancing. Even if I wanted to I couldn't help but tell this woman the truth. I told her about her panties and how her grinding had excited me.

"She seemed to like that and she asked me if I would like her to dance for me right then and there. She said I would have to pay but I didn't care. I would have gladly paid her everything I had.

"She slowly undressed, taking off everything but her panties. My heart was practically pounding out of my chest.

"While she was in her panties, she rubbed herself, thrusting her pelvis toward me. Then she danced out of her panties and held them out to me. She teased me with them, forcing me to beg for them. I crawled toward her on my knees.

"Then, laughing, she let me grab her panties from her. I immediately began to masturbate with them, coming quickly. She continued to laugh at me and she called me a fucking pervert. That's what she called me too, a fucking pervert.

"'Of course,' she said, 'I'm no angel myself. I like to take it up the ass. Do you like to give it up the ass?' She turned and pushed her ass into my face, spreading her cheeks. 'Would you like to put it up my ass?' She rubbed her ass at me, all the while telling me how she liked incredible sensations.

"Then she tied me up on the bed. Once my hands were tied, she stripped my clothes off until I was completely naked. She used her lips to kiss up my legs. She masturbated me with her breasts. Then she poured oil all over my penis and my ass.

"She stroked me while she put two, maybe three, fingers up my backside. Then she climbed up on me and slid my erection into her back door. Up and down she went, sliding me in and out of her while she masturbated.

"She orgasmed a number of times. Finally, she seemed exhausted. She untied me and told me I could go. I made sure that I took her panties with me when I left." Nathan lowered his head. "That wasn't all I left with obviously." He gestured toward his penis. "Now I've got all this to contend with."

To a great extent, Nathan's sexual preferences were very safe. The greatest danger to him was in his acquisition of used panties. Although anytime he behaved like a voyeur—a peeping Tom—he was invading an unsuspecting individual's privacy and running afoul of the law and so incurred the risks associated with that. However, as soon as Nathan engaged in sexual relations with a woman—and found himself engaged in a fairly high-risk type of physical activity—he was no longer in any kind of safety zone.

Unprotected anal intercourse outside of a monogamous relationship is a high-risk type of sexual behavior. Nathan discovered that the hard way. The biopsy that I performed on the warts on his penis, anus and legs showed that he had contracted venereal warts from his experience with the topless dancer.

Fortunately, these could be treated fairly readily. Nathan was grateful for that.

"What about the panties, doc?" he asked. "I can't catch

anything from them, can I?"

"The likelihood isn't great," I told him. "But it can't be dismissed. If you are pressing anything against you which has another person's body fluids on it, you run the risk of being exposed to disease."

I suggested that he wear a condom when he was masturbating with a pair of panties that were less than two weeks old. After that, I told him that the risk was fairly infinitesimal. He seemed quite relieved by that.

16

WHEN LOVE HURTS, AND THAT'S HOW HE LIKES IT

Rocco doesn't look like a man you'd associate with masochistic tendencies. Ah, but there's that reality again—*doesn't look like*. What are we to make of that observation. I have been forced to repeat it over and over again. This patient and that patient *didn't look like someone who* would suffer from an STD. This patient and that patient *didn't look like someone* who would engage in that type of sexual behavior. This patient and that patient *didn't look like someone* who would be so sexually active, or sexually "perverse", or sexually anything at all.

It is sometimes shocking to me how the public perception of sexuality is colored by the rantings and ravings (*that* is my editorial comment) of magazines like *Vogue*, or *Cosmopolitan*, or *People* or any one of a hundred magazines that you could identify easily. Our perception of sexuality is slanted by the actors and actresses that are presented to us in movies and on television. Even pornography (maybe *especially* pornography) distorts our "common knowledge" perception of sex and sexuality.

From the old days when "good girls don't" to our current days when sexual activity seems the sole province of women with "perfect" bodies (read, big breasts, narrow waists, long, smooth thighs) and men with equally "perfect" bodies (read, full head of hair, broad shoulders, well-defined abs, and a huge penis). It is small wonder that I was recently reading the newspaper and was astonished to learn about the remarkable increase in plastic surgery in young girls.

That older men and women are availing themselves of body sculpting is no longer news to anyone but that young girls not even firmly in the midst of puberty would undergo a surgeon's knife in the pursuit of physical perfection should cause all of us to take pause. Not only is the nature of "perfection" something that is open to various opinion but even if a person was able to attain that "perfection" it would be, by definition, temporal. It wouldn't last. And then what?

I remember, a number of years ago, I was watching one of those interview shows on television. The host, I believe it was Barbara Walters, was interviewing three women. Two of them were considered to be beautiful and were held up to be two of the sexiest women around. The third, remarkably talented and funny, was hardly what anyone was calling a beauty.

Ms. Walters concluded her interview with each of the women with the same question, which I will paraphrase. She asked each, on a scale of one to ten, to say how beautiful they thought they were. The two "beautiful" women acted predictably coy when asked the question. They expressed artificial humility and shyness. "Oh, my gosh, I don't know..." or something truly ridiculous like, "I don't think I'm all that pretty..." (which, curiously, probably *was* true).

After being prodded by Ms. Walters they each gave themselves some relatively high number, and eight or a nine. Then, Ms. Walters asked the same question of the third, un-beautiful woman. She looked Ms. Walters directly in the eye and without missing a blink she said, "Darling, I'm an eleven!"

Ms. Walters was flabbergasted. "But.. but.." Then, realizing she was being rude, she laughed with the guest. But, of course, the guest was serious. Beauty is a difficult concept indeed.

I have asked many patients to list for me the various sexual organs. Some are ignorant of any but the most obvious ones. When their answers are limited to the penis or the vagina, I restate my question. I ask them to list the various *sensual* organs that play an instrumental role in sexual arousal and pleasure. Sometimes the list grows more extensive after that. However, invariably, my patients leave out the one organ that I believe *must* be understood to be the primary sex organ—the brain.

It's a curious thing that the organ which is instrumental to arousal, pleasure, fantasy, and fulfillment is also the organ that filters and articulates perceptions of beauty and, even more curiously, is also the organ which holds the key to knowledge, the very knowledge which could allow each of us to enjoy *safe*, fulfilling, wonderfully pleasurable sex.

The brain.

Ah, but I have run far afield of Rocco. And, although Rocco might never have been the typical model for *People* magazine, he was a real person who came to me with a real problem.

He was presenting with blisters on his penis and a number of lesions, one in his mouth.

"I guess I should give you some idea how I got them," he said, referring to the irritations. "I mean, I know you're not a shrink or anything but I got to tell you a little about me. Maybe you'll understand then." He paused. He was clearly uncomfortable with the position he found himself in. "I.. I don't know if you want to hear all this crap..."

"No, please," I assured him. "I would like to hear what you have to say. I want to help you as best I can. I can't do that if I don't understand you. And," I added, "if you need additional help beyond what I feel capable of providing, I will be glad to recommend people I trust.

He smiled gratefully. The lines that had furrowed his forehead seemed to smooth out.

"I'm fifty-two years old," he began, almost apologetically.

I had the feeling that he felt that he shouldn't be coming to me for help at that age, that he felt, like most people that he should have just "grown up" and gotten over his needs. Maybe he was like a lot of people who felt that sexual desire should just stop after young adulthood, people who would be repulsed to think that their grandparents continued to enjoy healthy sexual relations.

I once had the opportunity to speak to a group of high school students. At the beginning of my presentation, I gave them a questionnaire. One of the questions was, "Do you think your parents still have sex?"

I could tell when each student came to that question because their expressions invariably changed and it was possible to detect a palpable revulsion in their manner.

I commented on the reaction I observed but I didn't focus on it. My topic was sexually transmitted diseases and that interesting digression was one I did not have ample time to explore.

Rocco seemed to feel that, whatever his particular desires, they should have ended long before the "ripe old age" of fifty-two. However, they clearly didn't.

"Doc, I get a real sexual charge out of receiving pain. I'm a masochist." He held his hands up in an apologetic manner. "I've been like this as long as I can remember. I was probably always like this. But I remember it really starting during the early days of my sexual experience.

"Geez, I couldn't have been more than fifteen or sixteen..." His expression took on a faraway quality. "My step-father had a bad drinking problem. Even during the best of times he wasn't a very patient guy. He was a lot worse when he'd been drinking.

"Anyone, one time I thought I was alone in the house and I was in the bathroom masturbating. I was reading this magazine... I didn't hear him come into the house. The next thing I knew, he was opening the bathroom door. `What the...?` he shouted, seeing me and what I was up to.

"He called me a sick fuck and started to hit me. You'd think I'd have lost my erection, wouldn't you?" He shook his head. "Not me. I won't say I *liked* him hitting me. It hurt and I was scared. He was a very strong man and he was really angry. He was smacking me really hard. But I can't say I didn't like it either. Not only didn't I lose my erection, I *came* while he was hitting me.

"Pretty weird, huh?" he asked, casting me a furtive glance. Then he shrugged his shoulders. "Ever since that time, I've always enjoyed mixing pain and sex."

He paused and looked down at his hands. "Anyway, to make a long story short, not too long ago I was bored and looking for some action. I don't have these masochistic experiences all the time. That would be too exhausting. But if too much time goes by between them I start to get antsy and itchy and all out of sorts.

"That's how I was feeling. Until very recently, I had a mistress named Teresa. She specialized in the kind of sadism that just drove me wild. I could always count on her to give me an experience that would leave me satisfied for days and days. She knew exactly how to treat her slaves, mixing humiliation and pain perfectly. But she got married and moved to California.

"I was in a panic. What was I going to do? She refused to give me to another mistress. That was her final punishment. I was going crazy until a friend of mine gave me the phone number of Mistress Monica.

"You can imagine how my fingers trembled when I dialed that number. I called and made an appointment right away.

"You'd have thought you were in a luxurious doctor's office. The reception area was wood paneled with deep, mahogany wood. A beautiful secretary handed me an application form to complete. `So the mistress will know what you are seeking,' she said with a knowing smile.

"I filled out every question and handed it back to her. She read over each response, sometimes glancing over at me with a knowing expression. Then she said I could wait in the main waiting area, that someone would be right with me. She pressed a buzzer and I walked through a door into a beautifully decorated room.

"The chairs were all leather. There were dark tapestries and fine paintings on the walls. I sat in one of the chairs and waited. I didn't have to wait long before the receptionist called me in. She directed me to a doorway.

"She told me to take my clothes off and then go through the door. I looked at her. `Here?' I asked. She looked at me sternly and nodded her head. She placed her hands on her hips and watched as I took off all my clothes. She eyed me up and down, clearly critical, then she motioned for me to go through the door. As I was walking through the door, she told me to wait on my knees.

"Inside the door were darkly-lit, seductive dungeons. Each was fitted with all sorts of gadgets and equipment particularly suited for this particular brand of pleasure. I was kneeling alone for a moment when a beautiful, blonde girl strode in.

"My God, you can't imagine the way I felt when I saw her. Mistress Naomi was wearing a leather dress, a garter belt, black silk stockings, no panties and, the thing that just sent shivers up and down my spine—six-inch stiletto heels.

"I reached out to touch her perfect flesh but she quickly smacked my hand away. `Dog,' she snapped. I started to beg her to let me touch her. She smacked me in the face and yelled at me that I was never to speak without permission."

The scene Rocco described became even more involved in this sad-masochistic game.

"Get on your feet!" the dominatrix commanded him.

When he scrambled to his feet, she stepped up to him and leaned into him so her face was inches from his. "You will obey me without hesitation, do you understand? You will do whatever I tell you to do because you know that I am the queen and you are just my pitiful slave. My toy. And if you hesitate I will crush you with my six-inch heels as you worship at my throne.

"Do you understand? Do you?!"

Rocco nodded meekly.

"You will submit completely to my superiority while I punish you mercilessly in my cell." She viewed him with disdain. "You are weak of heart and feeble of mind," she observed dismissively. She placed her hands on her hips. Then she lifted her right foot.

"Kiss my big toe," she commanded.

"Nothing will please me more," Rocco answered feebly as he fell to his knees and began to lick her toe.

"You can do better than that!" Mistress Naomi commanded.

Rocco licked more energetically.

"Suck it! Suck it like it's a penis!"

Rocco took her big toe in his mouth and began to suck on it. He was becoming more and more aroused when she withdrew her toe.

"You're a dog and I'm going to treat you like a dog." She placed a collar around his neck and tightened it.

As she pulled the leash, the collar squeezed his neck. Rocco began to gasp and beg for release. But Naomi didn't listen. Instead, she pulled the leash and dragged him over to a padded table. She forced him face down onto the table.

Still tugging on the leash with one hand, she took each of his hands with her other and strapped them high above his head. Then she walked around behind him. Spreading his legs, she forced a large object into his ass.

"Yes, you like that, don't you?" she asked as she thrust the object in and out of his ass.

She reached under him and felt his throbbing erection.

"Yes, you do, don't you?"

After a time, she withdrew the object. "You have earned your reward," she said. She called the name of another woman. Rocco could not tell if this woman worked at the academy or if she was another slave who was being called to do her mistress' bidding.

It didn't matter.

Naomi released Rocco's hands and pulled him up from the table. She led him over to a horizontal bar against the opposite wall. She strapped his hands onto the bar so that he was standing up with his hands high above his head. He was left facing the woman Naomi had called in.

Mistress Naomi walked around behind Rocco, the staccato of her heels echoing in the chamber. She waited several exquisite moments before he felt her hands on his ass again. Once again, she thrust a large object up him.

His erection began to throb.

"Suck him off!" Naomi commanded the other woman.

So, as she continued to thrust the object in and out of his, the woman sucked greedily on his penis until he experienced what he described as one of the most unbelievable orgasms of his life.

The woman giving him a blow job stood up and kissed him, her mouth filled with his semen. He kissed her back as she deposited most of his semen in his mouth.

A moment later, Naomi was releasing his hands from the bar. She pointed to his clothes in a pile by the door. Rocco kissed her on the feet. "Thank you," he said meekly.

He quickly dressed. On the way out, the blonde receptionist asked him to schedule his next session.

After he had finished telling me this tale, Rocco remained silent for several long moments. "And now I've got this," he said when he was finally ready to speak again.

Within five days of his encounter, the blisters had appeared on his penis. Shortly after, they became erosions.

"What's the matter with me, doc?" he asked plaintively. "I mean, I know what gets me off isn't normal but I've never had anything like this before. Am I being punished by God?"

I assured him that, to the best of my knowledge, God's judgment had nothing to do with his current suffering. My examination and subsequent culture indicated that Rocco had herpes genitalis.

Although there is no cure for herpes, there are a number of treatments which have proven to be helpful in minimizing the symptoms.

When I suggested to Rocco that he use a condom the next time he had any kind of sexual encounter in a non-monogamous relationship in which he knew his partner was disease free, he said that could never happen.

"I'm not allowed to make that kind of decision," he said.

"But, Rocco, it's possible that you could infect someone else now as well."

"I don't know what to do."

I suggested that he speak with a friend of mine who was a psychiatrist, a psychiatrist who worked with a lot of individuals with sexual issues. I explained to Rocco that I wasn't suggesting that he be "cured" of his sexual drives, whatever that might mean. Rather, I wanted him to be able to engage in his sexual preferences in a way that minimized the risk to himself and to others.

He agreed that he would make an appointment to see him.

17

SOMETIMES IT'S JUST A MATTER OF TRUST

One of the common—and I think, valid—criticisms of Freud is that he developed his psychology based on his many patients, all of whom exhibited marked neuroses. The criticism suggests that Freud's worldview was therefore skewed by the abnormal versus the normal. While I am not interested in being involved in a discussion of the problems of using the terms "normal" and "abnormal" in *any* context let alone a psychological one the underlying truth of the criticism is an observation that people generalize on what they know best. Freud happened to know neuroses best and so he generalized on them. In doing so, he offered some remarkable insights into the workings of the human psyche.

As a physician who treats patients suffering from sexually transmitted diseases, it is quite easy for me to view the world through the "rose colored glasses" of the activities of my patients. Recalling that many of my patients contract STDs through sexual activities which are contrary to vows of marriage and protestations of fidelity often makes me more accepting of the failings and foibles of people.

Because I am not at all shocked by the various ways in which my patients seek and receive sexual pleasure, I tend to be accepting of *any* activity which is pleasing to a person and which does not exploit or harm another person.

Like Freud, I generalize based on my knowledge and experience. While a large percentage of my patients have contracted STDs from adulterous sexual relationships—say seventy percent—statistics indicate that not nearly that many people engage in adulterous relationships.

My experience seems to indicate the statistics are off. Our culture is inundated with sex, with tales of adultery, of sexual prowess, of come-ons. As a result, we all tend to generalize. We often *presume* that "where there's smoke, there's fire."

We're not always right. Sometimes trust and faith should occupy a more honored place at our tables.

Marta, a sweet, thirty-five year old mother of three children, came to me not too long ago. With short, dark hair and a quick smile, she seemed to be the kind of person you would love to have as a neighbor.

"I see all kinds myself," she began. "I'm a dental assistant so you can imagine what I see. People, decent people who live in beautiful houses, come in with the most horrible teeth. Mostly it's bad hygiene. Sometimes it's genetics. Point is, you can never who's going to have bad teeth." She lowered her eyes. "I guess you can never tell who's going to have to come to you either," she added in a quiet voice.

I felt a tremendous sympathy for Marta. "Why don't you explain to me why you're here?" I asked her.

She colored slightly. "I.. I've been having some pain during intercourse," she said. "And I have a severe discharge." She made a face. "And it itches terribly."

"How long have you had these symptoms?" I asked.

"A few weeks ago, I started having some vaginal pain. It was a vague kind of discomfort. Intercourse made it a lot worse. Although my husband and I had sex a number of times I couldn't really enjoy it and I didn't have an orgasm at all."

She looked at me. "Do you think the birth control pills could have anything to do with it?"

"It's possible," I told her. "First we'll have to try and determine what's causing the discomfort..."

"The pain started about a week or so after Larry got back from a business trip," Marta said suddenly. Then her eyes filled with tears. "I can't believe he'd do something like this."

I looked at her curiously. "Something like what?" I asked.

She wiped her eyes and then blew her nose. "He must have gotten something when he was away on business. He must have given it to me," she complained.

"You suspect your husband had sexual relations with someone while he was away?"

"What else can it be?" she asked bitterly. "I mean, *I* haven't done anything outside our marriage."

We spoke a little while longer. She and Larry had been married—quite happily—for just over ten years. Although her hours were flexible to allow her to be available for the children, Larry tended to work long hours as a computer programmer.

"I always knew what that would be like," she explained. "Programmers are compulsive. They work on line after line of computer stuff. It's exhausting. I've always tried to make things easier for Larry."

"Have you spoken to your husband about your suspicions?" I asked her.

"Oh sure. Of course I did. I had to. He denied everything though. He said that he hadn't had sex with anyone else."

"You don't believe him?"

"I want to believe him," Marta said. "But then how do I explain what's going on with my body?"

"What about Larry? Is he exhibiting any symptoms?"

She seemed annoyed. "Of course he is," she said. "But you'd have to talk to him..."

"I think maybe I should. Regardless of what's going on, it seems that both of you will have to be treated."

"Well, he's out in the waiting room," she said, motioning with her head. "Have him come in if you want."

I buzzed my receptionist and asked her to have Larry join Marta and me in my office. When he came in, Marta turned a bit, offering him the cold shoulder. I got up and shook his hand. Larry, a thin, intellectual-looking man, smiled briefly.

"What is it?" he asked anxiously.

"Oh, you *know* darn well what it is," Marta snapped.

Larry looked at me apologetically. "I know what she thinks it is, doctor. But I swear, I didn't do anything wrong. I love my wife..." He turned and faced Marta. "I love you. I wouldn't do anything like that... and I trust you."

His shoulders sagged and he faced me. "I've been working an awful lot lately. I.. I haven't been able to show Marta the attention she deserves." He lowered his eyes. "Maybe she felt she had to turn to someone for affection..."

Marta wheeled around. "Oh, now you're trying to put the blame on me?" she said. "You've got a lot of nerve."

"I don't like to think so," he reasoned. "And it would be all my fault," he went on. "But..."

Anxious to cool the passions that were being tossed about in the office, I stood up and suggested that I examine both of them—separately. Only then could I begin to get to the bottom of the situation.

I discovered that Marta indeed had significant vaginal discharge along with irritation to the entire groin area. Larry's penis exhibited redness and he complained of itching and irritation of the head of his penis.

After taking cultures, I had them both dress and return to my office. I told them that I should know the result of the cultures within a couple of days. "Until then," I advised them, "refrain from sexual activity."

"Don't worry," Marta said, eyeing Larry suspiciously.

I gave them both a prescription which would alleviate some of the discomfort and promised to be in touch with them as soon as I got the results of their tests.

When I received their lab work the diagnosis was candidiasis in both cases. This, I felt, was an interesting finding in this situation. Vulvovaginal candidiasis is the most common form of vaginitis that is seen either in private practices or in clinics. Yearly, approximately three million women are treated for it.

What is most interesting about this disease in the case of Larry and Marta is that it is transmitted either sexually or *nonsexually*. While sexual transmission increases the bacterial colonization of the genitals, nonsexual transmission can be brought about by pregnancy, diabetes, antibiotics, systemic steroids, and *oral contraceptives*. Each of these conditions and/or medications alters the vaginal environment, allowing for a growth of the organism.

The organism itself is present in the normal flora of the vagina and coronal sulcus of the penis. In other words, *it's always there.* However, when conditions are normal and balanced, the organism is held in check. When there is an imbalance, the organism flourishes, resulting in the kinds of symptoms Marta and Larry exhibited.

The organism can be treated. The use of condoms are recommended during treatment in order to avoid the infection from being passed back and forth between the two partners.

"You mean I have a yeast infection?" Marta asked when I informed her of the lab results.

"Yes," I said.

"I.. I can't believe..."

I nodded my head to myself. I had allowed myself to jump to the simple conclusion that she had jumped to. Seeing so many cases of infidelity made such things presumptions rather than exceptions. Fortunately, there was an objective test that set us all to rights—and reminded me that in addition to tolerance a good dose of faith in one another is often well deserved.

18

WHEN SEX EQUALS DISEASE

Consensual, adult sex, regardless of the form the act takes, regardless of the gender and number of the partners, regardless of the nature of the relationship shared by the people engaged in it should be pleasurable. When disease, rather than pleasure, is the result, the sex act becomes a destructive act. In the United States today, thirteen million new cases of STDs effect men and women each year. In our young adult population, conservative estimates suggest that the total cost of STDs to society exceeds $2 billion annually.

The cost of gonorrhea alone exceeds $1.1 billion.

Clearly, in addition to the private hell that STDs represent in the lives of their victims they also add up to a significant public health issue. And it is in this realm, in the realm of public health, that sex and sexuality demands a public forum. *Not* in the ravings of conservative preachers, red-headed or otherwise. *Not* in the self-serving prattle of politicians. *Not* in the self-righteous proclamations of parents who have no idea what their children are really doing.

STDs have very real consequences in individual lives. They cause:

tubal pregnancies which may prove to be fatal to the mother and are *always* fatal to the unborn child;

death or severe birth defects to a baby born to a woman infected by any number of STDs;

sterility (the loss of the ability to become pregnant) in either men or women;

cancer of the cervix (a very real consequence for women who are very sexually active and/or who have STDs);

damage to other parts of the body, including the heart, the kidneys, and the brain, and;

death to infected individuals.

STDs are anything but a joke. And the most frightening thing of all is that they are becoming more and more difficult to treat. While some have eluded our ability to find a cure thus far others which we have believed were curable for years are now presenting in drug-resistant forms.

The growing complexity and incidence of STDs have required all of us who provide clinical care to employ the most current diagnostic and treatment methods. The Center for Disease Control (CDC), the Red Cross, and all the other public health organizations have responded to the growing incidence of STDs with a number of programs, both devoted to treatment and to education. Posters, pamphlets, vans, classes, and personal counseling interventions in schools are just some of the methods being used to address this public health crisis.

This book is part of my effort to address the need for education in confronting STDs. People—you—must realize that STDs are a very real danger that do not happen to the person in another part of the city, to the person of another ethnic or religious background, or to the person who makes less money than you do. STDs happen to your neighbor, to your friend, to your family member. STDs happen to YOU.

Only when that first level of defensiveness, the belief that you are immune to these diseases, has been erased, can you benefit from the humanity and human suffering shared in these pages.

While abstinence might be the best defense against STDs, it might also be the least practical. People have sex. Whether you believe it is right or wrong to do so is rendered irrelevant by the reality of it. That being the case, the next best defense is knowledge—and appropriate action taken because of that knowledge.

First and foremost, it is important for you to know exactly what is meant by the term, "sexually transmitted diseases". Clearly, they are diseases that are contracted through sexual contact. However, beyond that commonality, there is a broad range of diseases with a broad range of symptoms and possible treatments and outcomes.

Chancroid was, until recently, a disappearing disease in the United States. It has been reintroduced on the East Coast by immigrants from the Caribbean and on the West Coast by people from Mexico and Southeast Asia. The causative agents include hemophilus and ducrey. Incubation is between three and fourteen days in men. The primary lesion, a painful red papule or pustule, rapidly becomes puffier until it ruptures and forms an irregularly-shaped ulcer with excavated depth.

In women, the disease may be asymptomatic or there may be a painful ulcer that appears on the walls of the vagina and cervix.

Treatment *is* available and all patients should be seen a weekly intervals until a complete clinical cure is achieved.

Herpes is a viral disease. It produces groups of blister-like sores on the sex organs about two to 14 days after infection. Sometimes these blisters are accompanied by fever. The sores will break open and become painful especially if they come in contact with urine.

Although the herpes sores will disappear, the virus is still present and the sores can return without warning. Contagion through sexual contact is most likely when the sores are present.

Cold sores are also a form of herpes. People with sores on their mouths or lips should not have oral sex because this may cause genital herpes in their sex partners.

If you are pregnant and have genital herpes you should tell your doctor. If precautions aren't taken during childbirth, herpes can cause serious damage or even death to your baby.

Although there is no cure for herpes, there are a number of new drugs available which can minimize symptoms and discomfort.

Syphilis is caused by an organism that enters the bloodstream during sex and can attack all parts of the body. Within ten to ninety days after infection, a sore may appear on or around the sex organs, the rectum or mouth. This sore is painless and may be mistaken for a pimple or cold sore. *The sore will usually heal on its own in two to three weeks.* It may be followed by a rash, fever, headache, swollen glands, sore throat or sores in the mouth. *Or it may heal on its own with no additional symptoms.*

Syphilis can be treated with antibiotics but no medicine can repair the damage that syphilis has already done. Untreated, syphilis can cause blindness, heart disease and insanity. In a pregnant woman, untreated syphilis can cause birth defects and even death to her unborn baby. It is *very* important for pregnant women to have a blood test for syphilis as soon as they know they are pregnant.

Gonorrhea is caused by bacteria spread from one infected person to another during sex. It can attack the urethra in a man's penis, the cervix in a woman's vagina, and the rectum and throat. In men, the disease may cause burning during urination and discharge from the penis. Women *may have no symptoms* at all. They may not even know they are infected unless the disease if found during a routine examination.

This symptomless disease poses a particular danger because, untreated, it can cause sterility. In women, it can lead to Pelvic Inflammatory Disease (PID)—an infection which causes severe lower abdominal pain and fever, and can result in sterility or miscarriage.

Chlamydia (cervicitis) is an inflammation of the cervix caused by an organism passed during sex. Symptoms of this infection in women are mild but, when present, usually include a vaginal discharge. Untreated, chlamydia can cause pain, fever, miscarriage and infertility in women. Infants born to women with chlamydia can develop eye infections and pneumonia.

Non-gonococcal urethritis (NGU) is an infection which may cause burning upon urination and discharge from the penis. It is not caused by gonorrhea even though the symptoms are similar. It is usually caused by chlamydia and can be passed to partners during sex. Symptoms of an NGU infection can sometimes be so slight that the infected person may not even suspect an illness.

Hepatitis B is a liver disease caused by a virus carried in the blood, saliva, semen and other body fluids of an infect person. It is spread by sexual contact as well as several other means. Symptoms may include tiredness, poor appetite, fever, vomiting, joint pain, hives, rash or jaundice (a yellowing of the skin and the whites of the eyes). Doctors prescribe bed rest for those with hepatitis B. Most recover but some become long-term carriers of the virus and can spread it to others through sex.

<u>Venereal warts</u> are also caused by a virus and usually develop on the sex organs one to three months after exposure. Small warts are treated with medicine applied to the wart. Left untreated, the warts can spread or become so large that surgery is necessary. They can also bleed and become very painful.

The sexual partner of a person infected with venereal warts has about a 60% chance of getting them too. Women with venereal warts should have a yearly Pap smear because the virus has been linked with cervical cancer.

<u>Vaginitis</u> is an inflammation of a woman's vagina caused by tiny organisms that can be passed during sex.

<u>AIDS</u> is caused by a virus carried in the blood, semen and/or vaginal fluid of an infected person. Symptoms can include extreme tiredness, swollen glands, fever, night sweats, weight loss, a dry cough and diarrhea. The virus must get into your bloodstream to cause AIDS. This can happen during sex with an infect person or in any other activity in which body fluids are shared. A woman with the AIDS virus can give it to her unborn baby if she becomes pregnant

There is no cure for AIDS and in spite of the newer treatments the prognosis remains bleak.

Even this cursory review of a handful of the most prominent sexually transmitted diseases should be sufficient to convince you that you would want to take steps to *avoid* them.

19

IN SEARCH OF A FANTASY FULFILLED

There are many reasons that men and women find themselves in new sexual situations. Not all result from "dissatisfaction" with their current situation. There have been many, many times over the years that I have asked my patients to identify all the sexual organs they can name. Just as the resulting list inevitably includes penis, vagina, breasts, ass, etc. it just as inevitably fails to include the single most powerful sexual organ than any person has—the brain. More specifically, the mind and the imagination.

Long ago, I once heard a comedian compare marriage to Playboy magazine. The only difference being that "you get the *same* issue of the magazine" every single month for the rest of your life.

Implicit in the comedians joke was the need for variety. While a change in photographs suffice with magazines, for most people "variety" is created in their minds with their imaginations. Few things contribute to a successful sexual relationship as much as fantasies.

This is not to suggest that every fantasy must—or should—be fulfilled. For most people, it is the imaginative nature of the fantasy and the *possibility* of its fulfillment that contributes to sexual satisfaction. Indeed, like the difference between anticipation and fulfillment, fantasies fulfilled for many people can never come close to being what they had dreamed of. In other words, in the "real world" they lose their vibrancy and their color.

Maybe this is a variation of "the grass always being greener on the other side". That level of reflection is beyond the scope of these considerations. However, what is very much relevant for my patients is the possible consequences of fantasies fulfilled.

For a number of people, having their sexual fantasies realized opens a wide door of experience. It changes them, often for the better.

One thing remains certain, regardless of the positive or negative effects of a fantasy, fulfillment changes the participant.

That was certainly the case for one of my patients, a young (twenty-two years old) man named Sal. When he came to me, he explained a very common male fantasy.

"As long as I could remember I wanted to make it with two girls at the same time," he said to me, sitting across from me in my office. "I guess it started back when I was just twelve or thirteen. I was swimming at the public pool and two friends of mine, girls, were swimming around me. We were going under water, swimming under each other's legs and stuff. There was one point where they were both brushing against me and I had this big boner... I was wild. Embarrassed. Excited. Crazy. I went off swimming by myself until I calmed down.

"I never forgot that sensation though. God, how I wished

we were alone in the pool and we were naked..."

I listened patiently. Sal seemed like a friendly young man. He was expressive. Quick to smile. Full of emotion. Although his skin bore some scars from teenage acne, he was not bad looking. Not a "ladies man" by any conventional definition.

"And all the magazines—the porno ones—they were always showing two girls together or two girls with a guy. Wild.

"Anyway, I was going out with Nancy for about a year. We were very sexual. She was a good girl. You know, she went to church and all. She worked at the mall. But she was a wild girl in bed. She liked it a lot of different ways. She definitely wasn't shy.

"One day, we had just finished having sex and I was just rubbing her back and butt like she liked me to and I said something about this fantasy. I didn't say anything explicit or anything, just something general. And she just shot up and faced me.

"Her eyes were staring at me like I had two heads. She screamed at me. 'You want me to make it with a *girl*?' she spat out, real disgusted. 'You're fucking disgusting!'.

"I tried to calm her down. I told her no, no. I didn't want her to do anything disgusting. It was nothing. She wouldn't let it go though. I mean, she was all right that afternoon. But she kept bringing it up at weird times. Sometimes when we were out to dinner. If I looked at another girl, she got crazy. She'd ask me if that was a girl I was thinking of.

"It messed up our sex, I'll tell you. She got real... I don't know, squeamish almost. Things we always liked doing, she didn't want to do so much anymore. It was real weird."

"It sounds as though she was threatened by your fantasy,"

I noted.

"Yeh, I thought of that too," he admitted. "I kept telling her that I loved her and that I loved having sex with her. I tried to ask her about her fantasies. You know, maybe so she wouldn't feel so weird about mine. But she said she didn't have any fantasies."

"How can that be, doc?"

"She might not have been aware of her fantasies. Or, her fantasies could have been so frightening to her that she shut them out." I shrugged. "It's very difficult to know."

"Well, you can imagine that it wasn't long until we broke up. Jeez, I don't know how serious I was... but she just couldn't deal with me wanting to be with two girls together. Even if it was just in my mind. Even if she was one of the girls." He shook his head.

Sal went on to tell me that, in the next month or so after Nancy broke up with him, he happened to pick up a copy of Screw magazine.

"There was this *fantastic* layout of these two girls doing this guy. Just wild. They were *exactly* the kinds of girls I fantasized about. One even looked a little like Nancy, if you can believe that. The other one, the blonde, had this pussy that was just amazing... real plump, juicy lips. Man, my mouth got dry just looking at the pictures. And nice tits... not those real big floppy ones, but nice, tight ones. Unbelievable.

"When I continued looking through the magazine, I came to the ads in the back. One of them had a picture with it and the girl was the very girl from the layout. I can tell you what the ad said," he said, almost bragging. He recited the words: I am a hot and horny, single blonde. My juicy pussy's wet and ready. I'm anxious to meet a well-hung man whose into *anything!*.

"I kept that magazine for two weeks before I called. I was crazy with desire. You can't imagine. I beat off... masturbated... to that lay-out like three times a day. I was so turned on.

"Finally, I called her..."

With those words, Sal began to tell me the story that had direct bearing on his visit to my office. The first time he spoke to Lily, the woman in the ad, she spoke to him as if it were a typical, phone sex arrangement. However, he quickly explained that he was anxious to meet her.

"Why don't you come to my apartment?" she suggested.

"Are you sure?" he asked. Never having done anything like that before, he was a little uncertain about the "rules of the road".

Lily laughed. "Of course I'm sure. Why don't you come tomorrow afternoon? Oh, Sal, I *love* your voice. I'm getting wet just thinking about the things we can do..."

Sal arrived at Lily's apartment promptly at their agreed-upon time. Lily answered the door dressed in a sheer robe that covered a teddy and panty set. Sal could feel his heart pounding in his chest. He just stood in the doorway, staring at Lily. She was even more beautiful than she was in the photographs in the magazine.

"Umm," Lily sighed, giving him the once over. "You like just the kind of stud I love." She reached out and took his hand, bringing him into her apartment.

To Sal, she was everything he could imagine. She smelled like a flower. But more than a flower, she gave off the scent of sexual heat.

"Come in," she said, leading him into her apartment. "Come and sit down," she added, easing Sal down onto a nice, leather couch. "Can I get you something to drink?"

"Uh, maybe some beer," Sal said.

She smiled. "Okay, baby."

He watched her walk toward the kitchen. Her long legs and tight ass were magnificent. When she was gone, he looked around her apartment. It was really nice. The furniture was all modern. There were pictures on the walls. The king-sized waterbed dominated the bedroom.

Everything was a perfect combination of sexuality and elegance. He was blown away.

Lily came back with his beer. She handed it to him and then sat down next to him on the couch, pulling her long legs up under her. "So," she said, leaning toward him so that her robe opened and he could see clearly down the top of her teddy at her wonderful tits, "what is your fantasy?"

Sal sipped his beer. Finally, at the moment of truth, he found he had to calm the pounding of his heart to speak. "I.. I always wanted..."

She smiled and rested her soft hand on his knee. Slowly, she stroked his thigh, moving her fingers closer and closer to his crotch. "You can tell me, baby. Don't worry about a thing," she cooed.

"I.. I want to have sex with you and one of your friends," he blurted out.

She smiled. "Girlfriend?" she asked knowingly.

He nodded. "Yeh."

"Umm, I think that can be arranged," she said, her smile growing more seductive. She let her right hand rest just close enough to his penis that he could feel its pressure. Her left hand slowly teased the lacy material of her teddy. "I *like* your fantasy, baby." She leaned back. As she did, Sal was able to glimpse between her legs. He caught his breath at the brief sight of the pussy he had longed for.

"What kind of girl did you have in mind?" she asked, uncurling her long legs and standing up.

"Pretty like you," he said. "Like the one in the magazine," he added.

"Like Rachel?" she asked, nodding her head. "I love doing it with Rachel. Of course," she added, her voice becoming serious, "two of us will be a lot of money."

He told her not to worry. He had brought enough money.

"Good," she said. "I was hoping this would be a long afternoon as soon as I heard your voice yesterday. You made me so wet with your voice," she added. To demonstrate just how excited she was, she slipped her finger inside the lace of her panties. Moving it around languidly, she clearly found her mark, slipping it inside her sex. Her eyes closed and a wanton look came over her as her legs swayed side to side. A moment later, she withdrew her finger and slipped it between her lips. "I hope Rachel can come right over," she said in a soft voice.

Lily went to the phone and dialed a number. "Hurry," she said in a breathless, whispery voice. When she hung up, she turned to Sal. "Rachel's on her way. She won't be more than a few minutes."

When Rachel arrived, Sal grew light-headed. Rachel *was* the girl from the magazine. In person, she looked even more like Nancy, making the fantasy that much better. The difference was that Rachel had an even better body than Nancy and she had the most seductive eyes.

"Hi," she said when she saw Sal. "Lily told me you were a stud but she didn't tell me how much of a stud you really are," she said, smiling and running the tip of her tongue over her full lips.

She slipped out of her coat, revealing that she was wearing only a strapless tee shirt and bikini panties. She walked closer to Sal, who was still sitting on the couch. She slipped her hands inside the waistband of her panties and, as her fingers danced under the thin material, she formed a kiss with her lips.

Lily came up behind Rachel and stroked her shoulders with her hands. Slowly, she brought her hands around and cupped Rachel's breasts, pinching her erect nipples through the soft material of the strapless tee shirt. Rachel leaned her head back and met Lily's lips.

As Sal sat on the couch, staring at the tableau these two beauties were playing out before him, Lily and Rachel engaged in a long, soulful tongue kiss. When they broke it off, Rachel, looking flushed, looked Sal directly in the eye. "Oh, baby, I think we need to start moving to the bedroom..."

Both Rachel and Lily reached out to Sal to help him up. He hesitated for a moment. Now that his fantasy was to become a reality, he felt a sense of apprehension.

Rachel smiled knowingly. "Oh, don't be shy, baby. I'll show you everything you need to do." Then she took Lily's hand and guided it into her panties. As she kept her eyes on Sal, Rachel enjoyed the feel of Lily fingering her. Suddenly, she drew in a sharp breath. "Oh, baby, let's get to the bedroom before my knees give out."

Although Sal had a difficult time standing, what with his erection, he let the girls pull him up.

They both smiled at the hard bulge in his pants.

"I knew you weren't really nervous," Rachel said, reaching out and pressing her palm against his crotch.

The girls walked ahead of him to the bedroom, sashaying their marvelous asses and holding hands. Sal stopped in the doorway of the bedroom. Standing at the foot of the bed, Rachel slipped Lily's robe off her shoulders. Then she pinched the hem of Lily's teddy blouse and began to lift it up. Lily raised her hands up into the air as Rachel drew the satiny material up over her flat belly and then over her firm breasts. A moment later, Lily was standing in just her panties. Her nipples were erect.

Rachel leaned toward Lily and kissed her full on the lips. As she pressed herself against her, she slid her hands along Lily's bare back and under her panties, massaging her firm ass cheeks.

The two girls ground their pussies against each other. When they separated, Sal could see the moisture that had formed between their legs.

Rachel used the tip of her tongue and licked along Lily's neck. She kissed both nipples, pausing to suck them. Then she kissed her way down Lily's flat stomach. When she reached the waistband of Lily's panties, Rachel slipped her fingers inside the waistband and drew them down Lily's long legs.

Lily stepped out of the flimsy material even as Rachel remained, her lips and tongue locked between her legs. Lily let her eyes close. She rested her two hands on the back of Rachel's head and eased her tighter against her crotch.

"Umm," Rachel sighed, standing up. She eased Lily back onto the bed and pushed her knees open. She glanced at Sal. "Doesn't she have the most beautiful pussy in the world?" she asked, opening the folds of her thick lips.

Sal could only nod his head in breathless anticipation.

Rachel crawled onto the waterbed. Rocking slowly with the movement of the water, she pulled her sleeveless tee shirt over her head, exposing modest-sized tits capped with the loveliest nipples Sal had ever seen.

Then she slid down Lily's body and started licking Lily's cunt again. As she did, Lily pulled Rachel's panties off and began to lick her. The girls were moaning. The sounds of their slurping and moans were making Sal crazy. He continued to watch these goings on for only a couple of minutes and then he undressed and joined the girls on the waterbed.

"I was wondering when you were going to show up," Rachel said with a seductive smile. She turned her attention away from Lily for a moment and reached into his underwear to pull out his hard cock. "Oh, baby," she sighed, blowing on it before slipping the head between her lips.

Lily came around on the bed and began to lick his balls while Rachel sucked his pole. Soon, he was moaning. Rachel squeezed his dick.

"Not yet, baby," she cooed. "I want it up my ass first. I love the incredible feelings of taking it up my ass," she added, pressing her ass against his face as she said it.

Sal pressed his nose into the crack of Rachel's ass. He stuck out his tongue, wanting to taste anything and everything. She pushed her ass back harder as his hands began to explore her, a finger rubbing her asshole while another from his other hand toyed with her clit.

"Oh, baby, you know I like *that*!" she sighed. Then, to his disappointment, she eased away from him.

She and Lily laid him flat on his back.

"Don't worry about a thing, darling," Lily said. "You let us do all the work."

Rachel reached into the night stand and brought out some coconut oil. She poured the oil over his cock, rubbing it in, massaging it into his balls, reaching under him and fingering his asshole. He was soon jerking his hips, wanting to land his cock anywhere warm and tight.

Rachel straddled him. She reached behind her and grasped his erection. Holding it steady, she slowly eased herself down, impaling herself with his cock.

"Oh God, oh God," she whispered, her eyes closed as she felt the length of him going up her ass. "Oh yes..."

She began to move slowly up and down. As she did, she fingered herself.

Sal watched his cock disappearing into Rachel's ass and he thought he'd lose it completely. But then Lily began rubbing her beautiful tits against his chest and kissing him hard on the mouth. He could hardly breath.

There was one point when he thought to himself, This is it! I'm having two girls at once!

His fantasy was everything that he dreamed of. With Lily kissing him and Rachel riding him, he would have happily died then and there. Rachel started moving faster. A few moments later, as she screamed out in ecstasy, he came for the first time in her ass.

The afternoon didn't end there. In fact, that was just the beginning in a long session of fantastic sex. He ate Lily while she blew him. He sucked on Rachel's tits while Lily ate Rachel. When he was tired, he watched as they ate each other in a beautiful 69 position. They sucked him off together as he fingered them. He fucked Lily while Rachel sat on her face.

"What a circus it was!" he said to me, some of the emotion of that afternoon still in his voice. "I must have come six times! It was definitely worth having Nancy leave me!

"There was cum all over the place. The sheets were soaking wet with their juices and sweat. It was crazy. Their moans were real, doc. Not porno movie acting. It was the real thing.

"Of course, I understood that even fantasies have to come to an end. They each gave me a sweet kiss and then I paid them for a great afternoon of sex." He lowered his eyes. "I paid all right. And now I'm paying some more."

I looked at him curiously. "How so?"

"About two weeks after I was with them, I started having this drip from my dick. A gray color. Especially in the morning. And it itches like hell, doc. Christ, I can't believe I told those girls we'd have to do it again sometime. Not if I have to suffer like this!"

My examination and subsequent culture of the discharge showed that Sal was suffering from trichomoniasis. Fortunately for him, I was able to treat him easily. His fantasy had been a wonderful experience for him.

He suffered a STD that was treatable.

"I'm going to see if I can get back together with Nancy," he told me when he came in for treatment. "I mean, the fantasy was great but... well, I miss her..."

The needs of the body are demanding. So are the needs of the heart.

20

TEACHERS AND STUDENTS

There are many relationships that seem to invite the possibility of sexual contact. Indeed, any relationship in which there is any consistent contact holds the potential for intimacy but there are some which are especially "dangerous." The doctor-patient relationship is one. As is the psychologist-patient relationship. As powerful as these relationships are, they seem not to hold a candle to the power of the teacher-student relationship when it comes to the blossoming of sexual encounters.

Even when the student and the teacher are in relationships they are comfortable with, there is the heightened possibility of sexual encounter. When one of the two is "out of comfort" then the balance can tip dangerously in the direction of an illicit sexual relationship.

That was the case for one of my patients, Marsha.

Marsha, a very attractive woman of thirty-three, found herself "out there" as she put it, after her husband left her.

"Not that our relationship was so perfect," she noted with a touch of irony. "I mean, obviously, right? Robert was always a bit weird. A partyer. He'd drink too much. Some recreational drugs." She shrugged. "Not a big deal. I mean, we were young. No kids. We ran with an artsy crowd. There was no right and wrong. Not in the conventional sense. We were all selfish.

"Still, it was fun for a while. Then it got unpleasant. He said I was too inhibited. I couldn't let myself go..." She laughed softly to herself. "I guess I showed him, huh?"

I smiled briefly, hoping to put her at ease. She clearly came from comfortable circumstances and, as a musician, was involved in arts and, as she put it, had artsy friends. She played several instruments. These days, she found herself supporting herself by giving piano lessons in her home.

"According to the divorce settlement, Robert's supposed to send me alimony payments. But he's a musician too. When he works regular gigs, he generally sends along the money. When he doesn't, he can't. Fairly simple, huh?" She sighed. She adjusted her short skirt and then straightened the buttons on her simple, white blouse.

Her brown hair was cut short. She had lovely, dark eyes and a quick smile.

"Anyway, when Robert left, I just went on a tear."

"A tear?" I asked, not sure what she meant.

"Well, he wasn't wrong about my being inhibited," she said. "Of all the people we knew, I was probably the most conservative. I stayed away from drugs and I liked my sex simple. Me and Robert. Some foreplay. Missionary position." She spat out these terms as though she was challenging me. "Nothing kinky."

"And?"

"And all that changed after Robert left. I guess I was angry so I thought I'd... you know, show him. But then, I realized that he'd been right. I *was* inhibited and I didn't want to be like that any more.

"Call it the flip side of repression but I was completely out of control. If it had two legs and a dick, I'd have sex with it." She colored slightly after that statement. Although she had been, as she put it, on a tear for a while it was clear that the personality make-up that had made her the most conservative in her crowd was still very much in evidence.

"I guess I wanted to make up for lost time," she said, her voice growing a bit softer. "If it was something I'd have said no to in the past, I said yes to it. One time, I even got into some bondage." She let out a low breath. "That was a little weird. Getting tied up naked on the bed and getting knocked around." She rolled her eyes. "Nothing too violent. You'd be amazed at how strict the bondage rules can be." She studied me for a few moments. "Maybe you wouldn't. You've probably heard some wild stories..."

"You're not the first patient who has came into my office," I noted with a wry smile, wanting to put her at ease.

"I only did the bondage thing with this one guy—a real sleazebucket of a lawyer. He liked to slap and pinch me. He liked biting too. I still have some bruises and teeth marks." She gave an involuntarily wince. "He bit my nipple so hard once it started to bleed.

"I still have some bruises from him. Bastard," she added under her breath.

"Needless to say, I also ran through a bunch of musicians. Most of them I did because I wanted it to get back to Robert. Let's see," she went on, glancing upward as if she was doing a tally in her head. "Then there was the furniture salesman. An accountant I met in Martinique..."

She lowered her eyes and looked at me. "I was unstoppable. I was like an alcoholic. An addict. You name it, I did it. I couldn't be satisfied because the high wouldn't last. As soon as my body came down from one set of orgasms, I craved more. I wanted more. More.

"I grew desperate. I needed to have orgasms like drug addicts need to have their fix. I mean, the thought of making it with another woman had always appalled me... I'd fooled around with a dildo, like everyone else, but to actually *make it* with another woman... that was a little scary. That was crossing a line I wasn't ready to cross."

She leaned back into the chair and sighed. "There have been so many partners. Even in the past month." She looked me dead in the eye. "I couldn't tell you who caused what or when." She laughed aloud, as if anticipating something that I might be planning to say. "And safe sex? Forget it. I couldn't be bothered. I was an addict playing Russian roulette.

"Call it the gambler in me..."

As I listened to Marsha, I couldn't help but reflect how human sexuality so often holds a mirror up to our worst tendencies as well as it does to our best. While sex can mirror our sense of intimacy, of love, it can also mirror desperation and destructiveness.

Wanting to be physically satisfied is reason enough to engage in sexual behavior. However, engaging in a game of "Russian roulette" with one's health and well-being is indicative of a destructiveness that needs to be addressed in its own right.

However, one step at a time. Marsha had come to me with specific symptoms that would have to be addressed. I would help her to deal with the other aspects of her behavior, the aspects that contributed to the situation she was in, when it was most appropriate.

"The best," she went on, "was when I was teaching piano." She stopped. "Best? Well, yes. I guess, in a manner of speaking." She raised her eyes to mine. "I do have some scruples, doctor. I make it a policy not to have relationships with my students. I have to be *very* careful about that. It is my profession and my primary source of income.

"Not that I didn't fantasize about any number of them. Even so of the young girls. But there is this one student... he isn't young. He's about twenty-two. A college student. An engineering student. Very handsome. Sure, I'd *thought* about it but I had my rules.

"But then, I don't know what it was, something he said or did... I don't know. Maybe I was helping him with a particular piece and I had to sit on the bench beside him and lean toward the music to point something out. Maybe his arm brushed against my breast. Maybe it was the feel of him so close to me." She shrugged. "Maybe it was because it was a beautiful day. Who knows?

"The next thing I knew, I was glancing at his crotch and getting a little bit aroused." She paused. "When I'm aroused, my nipples get very erect. I don't usually wear a bra—just camisoles under my blouse—and it's possible to see my nipples.

"Anyway, my glances lingered a little longer. My nipples started to ache, rubbing against the material. I'm sure he must have seen the way I was reacting. Even though I did try to keep myself under control... but it was a losing battle, I'll tell you that.

"I could feel myself flush. I was getting wet... oh God, I was just losing control. But I didn't make the first move. He did.

"I was still sitting beside him on the bench and he turned and he just kissed me, full on the lips." She drew in a deep breath. "I normally would have slapped him. I should have slapped him. But this time... I couldn't help myself. I let him kiss me.

"Well, one thing led to another and... well, it wasn't long before we were naked... I'll give him credit for working quickly. Once he decided what he wanted, he got it. Determined fellow," she said, almost amused by the recollection.

"We did it on the couch near the piano. It was funny, you know. I mean, not funny ha ha, but funny strange, you know, getting screwed by one of my students. I mean, part of me was aware that *this was really happening*! I knew that the piano lesson was over for the day.

"Not that I couldn't have given him some other lessons. He didn't have much technique. He had a nice cock but nothing exceptional. Still, I enjoyed it very much.

"We did it a couple of times that afternoon. I even let him ejaculate in my mouth." She smiled. "I told him that it tasted like licorice."

Her shoulders sagged and she glanced down at her skirt. "So, doctor, I can't tell you exactly where I got all this crud from. Sure, I could quote Claude Rains from "Casablanca" and suggest we round up the usual suspects. But that wouldn't do any good.

"I don't even know half of them.

"If you ask me if I feel guilty, the answer is no." Then she looked at me with just a hint of suspicion. "I mean, it's not like I've got something you can't fix... do I?"

"I would hope not," I answered truthfully. "But I can't

know definitely until after an examination and some lab work. But, based on the description you've given me regarding your symptoms—the thin, grayish-white discharge, the itching, and the fishy-like odor, I would think that your STD is treatable."

As it turned out, Marsha was not suffering from an STD at all. The lab work showed that she was suffering from bacterial vaginitis. I was able to successfully treat her with an antibiotic.

"Thanks, doc," she said, grateful for my help.

"I'm glad to help, Marsha. I would like to discuss with you your decisions regarding engaging in unsafe sex..."

She frowned. "I thought you were non-judgmental," she said.

"I try to be," I told her. "And I would not question your sexual choices. However, I do feel the need to discuss with you practices that are harmful—or potentially harmful—to you. You seem determined to hurt yourself, Marsha," I noted, softening my voice.

Her eyes welled up. "I'm not happy about how things have turned out," she said. "You don't think I'm happy about all this, do you?"

I shook my head. "No, I don't think that at all."

"I was so hurt when Robert left..."

"Maybe the fact that you broke one of your own rules—having a sexual encounter with a student—is a sign that things have gotten a little out of hand."

She nodded. "I always told myself that would be the worst..."

"Perhaps we can discuss your decisions regarding your sexual relations... and maybe it would be beneficial if we were to include someone who might be able to help you get some perspective on your life and all your decisions."

Marsha clasped her hands in her lap and nodded. "Yes," she said in a quiet voice. "That would probably be a very good idea."

Too many people have trouble finding a balance when it comes to sexuality. For them, any expression of sexuality outside some very narrow "normal" is a significant deviation. Perhaps that means sex only in marriage with a spouse. Perhaps it means that, even under those circumstances, it means only genital-genital coitus in a missionary position. There are others who believe that sexuality is just a physical expression, an appetite, which must be sated. For them, there is no moral or emotional component to sexual expression.

While people with beliefs on either end of this spectrum are free to cling to those beliefs, my own medical experience suggests that either "misses the boat" when it comes to sexuality as an expression of human experience.

While there are a great many people who look for sexual outlets in many places, "sexual deviation" is a definition that is determined by another, arbitrary, definition—"sexual normalcy". Ultimately, deviation is simply that which is not "normal". If a particular society or culture defines sexual normal as being man and wife, within the bounds of marriage, only engaged in genital-genital intercourse then there exists a *very* broad spectrum of deviation. If "normal" is not nearly so narrowly defined then, by extension, deviation is not nearly so evident.

As long as sexual expression is not forced upon another individual, as long as it does not result in injury and real pain, as long as it involved only individuals old enough and mature enough to knowingly engage in it then it is "normal". Which is not to say it is not driven by negative impulses.

Marsha is a prime example. She was unhappy. For her, sexuality was a weapon of self-destruction, one over which she seemed to have very little control. No one who spoke with Marsha could come away from that conversation without realizing the negativity of her sexual choices. Her *intent* was wrong. However, the choice she made were not.

However, we are well-advised to remember that sexuality—as a human expression—is an emotional involvement (even short-lived). There are issues of trust and intimacy.

Sexuality in humans, is not like sexuality among certain animals. It draws into it the full range of humanity—religious beliefs, societal mores, emotional needs, physical needs, the sense of self and the desire to connect with another human being. There is nothing insignificant about all that—even if there are certain sexual adventures which seem not to call into account the full range of all this.

This should not be surprising. After all, there are meals we eat "on the run" and other meals we linger over. Meals which are like feasts and others which are little more than snacks. Meals we share with family and other meals which we eat in the company of strangers.

In all cases, we need nourishment. In most cases, we enjoy the meal more if we like what we're eating.

Some people eat in a destructive manner. That doesn't mean they don't need food. It only means that other considerations should be taken into account when considering those people.

It is like that with sex as well.

21:

THAT LOCKER ROOM SYNDROME

There is an old saying, "If you're talking about it, you're not doing it." That is very true regarding sexual experience. I've never been a fisherman so "fish stories" are not familiar to me. But I have heard thousands upon thousands of sexual adventures. The majority of them are honest and true. Why wouldn't they be? After all, by the time they get to me they aren't about bragging but about decisions that resulted in disease—sometimes fatal disease. It's true that, for the most part, descriptions of sexuality tend to be exaggerated. Breasts seem always to be firm and perfect. Penises are always extremely large and hard. Stomachs are always flat. Partners are always attractive. Unless, of course, the teller is angry or bitter. Then there is *nothing* right about the partner. They are clumsy. Inexperienced. Small. Flat. Fat. Too fast. Too slow.

You get the idea.

To a great extent, I listen to these details only as imperfect clues into the experiences of my patients. However, sometimes the gulf between the story I'm told and the truth is a very broad one—a veritable Grand Canyon.

That was the case with Sanford, a successful entrepreneur. When he came into my office, he looked at me in a very sheepish way. If you would have seen him on the street, you would not have suspected him of having an STD.

Sanford, at forty-two, was very overweight. His hair was thinning. His skin was oily and shiny. And, as for his emotional presentation... he was distraught.

"Doc, you've got to help me," he began, leaning forward in the chair. "I'm in a real pickle..."

I nodded. "Tell me what's going on," I urged him.

He drew a deep breath. "I was on vacation with my wife in Madeira," he began, his voice seeming to take flight at the mere mention of the place. "God, it was beautiful, doc. The sky was so goddamned blue... seemed to go on forever. Anyway, we were in the hotel and my wife was tired so she said she was going to take a nap. I told her that was fine, that I might go down by the pool. She didn't seem to care. A few minutes later she was snoring away. So, I went down to the pool. I figured I had a few hours to kill so, what the hell? Normally, I hate being outdoors. Give me a desk and a telephone and I'm in heaven... stick me outside and I'm out of my element.

"It was damned hot by the pool, I'll tell you that. And everywhere I looked, the women were topless. It completely blew me away. Now, I might be over forty but there's still a lot of the adolescent in me and I just couldn't believe all these women walking around with their tits hanging out.

"Of course, I don't want to look like a complete idiot.. you know, a gawking American tourist. I really wanted to get into that European thing. That.. you know... disinterested bit. I even had a beret. I thought I looked a little European.... no? Well, you should have seen me there," he said

"Anyway, when I got down to the pool, there was this one woman who really set me off. Now, I should explain," he went on, his voice dropping to a conspiratorial whisper, "I had my share of side action. In my line of work, it's almost expected. So, it's not like I wasn't hoping that something would happen.

"But I had to be discreet. Not only did I want to get the European thing down but my wife was upstairs in our hotel room, sawing some logs.

"At least, I wanted to be discreet. I don't know how well I managed that. Jesus, doc. This lady was unbelievable. About forty. Big, fat tits all greased up and soaking up the sun. *Everything* about her was big. She had a big belly, and a big ass to match her big tits. Huge thighs. The works. God, I was in heaven. Slop heaven. And those goddamned cool Europeans. Sitting by her and acting like she was wearing a bearskin coat instead of a little thong bikini thing and nothing else. Not me, I was thinking, *How can I fuck this baby?* I know that's what they were thinking too but they were playing it so goddamned cool...

"My mind was racing and my pants were heating up. What could I do?

"You can't imagine the things that went through my mind. Christ, doc, I even considered walking past her and spilling my drink on her! Can you imagine? How desperate would that have made me look?

"Do you appreciate the dilemma I was in? I couldn't very well just walk up to her and say, `Hi, I'm Sanford and I really, *really* like your tits. Would you like to fuck me?'

"In the end, I decided to play it the European way—cool. Hey, I'm a successful guy and I'm used to getting my way. And there's more than one way to skin a cat, right? I plotted out my strategy like it was a chess game..."

Sanford went on to describe in detail the way he'd maneuvered himself into a favorable position to watch this woman and then, slowly, as the sun shifted in the sky, he moved closer and closer to her until he was next to her.

"From there," he said, giving me a wink, "I was in like Flint!"

He seemed transported back to his vacation in Madeira as he described in passionate detail the sexual adventured he'd enjoyed with this woman. She was, it seemed, everything anyone could ever have desired. A fantasy fulfilled. She was able to bring him to orgasms so easily and then to coax his erection back in no time at all. They engaged in oral sex, anal sex—a regular Kama Sutra of different positions and sensations.

His descriptions were vivid and, as he spoke, it was possible to see how much he enjoyed reliving this passionate episode in his life.

There was only one problem. None of it happened. Not in Madeira. Not ever.

As it turned out, Sanford's reason for visiting me had a much more common explanation, one which he had been loathe to share with me. Unfortunately, the truth, for him, was a bit more humiliating.

Sanford was not a successful entrepreneur at all. He was an unemployed actor.

"Hell, I've never even been to Madeira," he admitted, his voice dejected. "I'd like to go though," he said, brightening up momentarily.

"Would you like to tell me what really happened?" I asked him.

"My goddamned girlfriend," he spat out. "Oh, I'm not married either," he added, almost as an afterthought. He looked me in the eye. "I'm not having any goddamned luck," he said. "That bitch, she's been having all the fun. Some relationship I'm in. She fucks everything and anything that moves... okay, I'm exaggerating. I guess that's a problem I have, huh? But she did my best friend. I'm sure about that. Probably only once or twice. I can't be sure. But I know it happened.

"And now look at me!

"Three days ago, I found out what a fucking bitch that whore really is. I got these tiny blisters all over my dick, on my thighs and on my butt. Doc, I'm going crazy at night with the itching, especially when I get overheated. And look," he went on, extending his hands toward me, "look at this crap between my fingers!"

As my examination revealed, Sanford had gotten herpes genitalis.

While the particular disease could be addressed, I came away from my meeting with Sanford very disturbed. The extent that he tried to disguise the truth about his sexual relationship was very disheartening.

The reality was that I was no more impressed by the story he was trying to get me to believe than I was disapproving of the truth. But he, like so many others, felt the need to present their sexual exploits in the most impressive terms.

One of the messages that I try to convey to my patients, in addition to the specifics of safe sex, is that good sex is not a function of size, stamina, weight, height, hair color, or any of the other things that we assign to "sexual appeal". Remember, the most potent sexual "organ" is the mind, the imagination. *That* is where the sex gets really good.

So many people struggle with their sexual identities for so many reasons, it seems tragic that deceit has to be a constant.

22

WHEN THERE'S NO SEX AT HOME

One of the presumptions of a happy marriage is that the sexual relationship between husband and wife is satisfactory. Unfortunately, for a number of reasons, this proves not to be the case. Now, I should quickly point out that "satisfactory" here is tremendously variable. What is "satisfactory" for one couple might not be for another. All that is necessary is that the level of sexual activity, its variation, and its intensity be satisfying to both partners.

When it is not—for whatever reason—the stage has been set for trouble.

This is what happened to Michael. At thirty-eight, he is a successful Wall Street broker who, due to the nature of his career, must work long, hard hours. Often times he does not know in advance when a particular deal will require him to work late into the night or on the weekends.

"Look," he said to me. "I know it's tough for my family as well. I come home late at night, sometimes after my two kids are already asleep. I can count on one hand the number of dinners we all have together in any given month.

"I wish it wasn't so tough for everyone. But, damnit, everyone sure likes what my hard work brings, don't they?" He went on to describe the material benefits of his job—the cars, the big house, the huge yard, the private schools. "No one complains about any of that," he noted with some bitterness. "I guess I should be flattered that they miss me in the house but if they had to trade my being there for the house itself... I'd guess they'd take the house."

That assessment might have been self-serving.

"Even with the long hours, things used to be a lot better. Look, I know it's not easy to be home with kids. But my wife has help. It's not like she's got to do the laundry and clean the house and take care of the kids... we've got a housekeeper and a nanny. She plays tennis and goes out to lunch with her friends... she's got it pretty easy if you ask me.

"I don't want to sound bitter, doc. I'm not. I mean, things were good with my wife and me. And she's good looking. That means a lot to me. Call me shallow, but I like my wife being beautiful. She used to wait up for me no matter how late I came home.

"God, sometimes we'd have these dirty conversations over the phone—I'd have the cell phone and she'd be waiting for me in bed... doc, it was unbelievable. But then, after our second baby was born, something changed. Cindi stopped paying any attention to me. When I came in late, she'd be in bed, snoring.

"She still looks good. Why shouldn't she? She plays tennis, goes to aerobics classes, has a personal trainer. The works. But after Willie, our second, it was like I was nothing but a paycheck. Our sex life went right down the drain. She was always tired. Or not in the mood. Or feeling bloated.

"Not that it was just her fault. Look, I work like a dog. There are plenty of times when I get home that I'm just beat. It's all I can do to wash my face before I collapse in bed. But... but it wasn't right what was happening. Wasn't right at all.

"When I tried to talk to her about it, you know, about not having sex for like a couple of months at a time, she just said that sex wasn't that important to her anymore. Her children are her priority.

"Hell, doc, I love my children too. I love my wife. We're married. That means something to me. But I'm a man, goddamnit. I have needs." He ran his fingers through his still-thick, dark hair.

"Anyway, I had to take this business trip to Puerto Rico. Two weeks. I never liked being away for so long but... I really needed to get away. Even if it was a business trip, I needed to be away. I just had to unwind. The couple of weeks before I left just seemed to be one fight after another with Cindi.

"So the time away couldn't have come at a better time. I stayed in a very nice, very comfortable hotel on the beach. The weather was just unbelievable. Warm. Sunny. Great. Every morning I went out onto the beach and went for a swim.

"The feel of the warm water just made me feel young again. Alive. I would let the sun dry me and then I'd go back to my room to shower and get ready for work. At the end of the work day, I'd come back to the hotel and go to the bar where I'd enjoy a shot of cognac and just people watch.

"It was nice.

After the first couple of days, I noticed a very attractive woman who would come into the restaurant by herself. She was probably about thirty. Really nice looking but not nice looking like a prostitute. You know what I mean? She didn't look like anything had been surgically enhanced or anything.

"Still, I couldn't figure out why such a beautiful woman would be alone. Maybe she *was* a prostitute, right? I mean, what did I know?

"Well, this one evening, she was in the bar just nursing a drink. I kept watching her out of the corner of my eye, wondering what she was about. I was damned curious, I'll tell you. Not that I expected anything to come of it. Jeez, not at all. But, like I say, I was curious.

"I decided that I would find out something about her. I just didn't know how. Then, the next evening, when she was seated in the same place, wearing a low-cut, very elegant evening dress—man, I was knocked out by how good she looked. Her breasts were just... just magnificent. As I would find out later, she wasn't wearing a bra.

"Anyway, I got up the courage to introduce myself. I slid off my barstool and started to walk over to her... right when the waiter was bringing her another drink. I bumped into him and the drink spilled on her dress. God, did I feel like a jerk. I couldn't apologize enough. I offered to buy her another drink. To pay for the cleaning of her dress. Anything. She was very sweet. She declined my offers. She was very gracious about it. She finally laughed and told me that it was all right, I could stop apologizing.

"We had met.

"Her name was Elissa. She was divorced and on the islands to get away. I told her about my own situation, that I was married, worked on Wall Street..."

As Michael spoke, Elissa listened closely. "Oh," she said when he told her about working on Wall Street. "Then you live in the City?"

"Yes," he said. "I live in the East 60s. Do you know the City?"

She laughed. "Of course. We're practically neighbors. I live in Short Hills, New Jersey."

They continued to talk, drinking champagne and enjoying the dying light of the evening. When she got up to leave, Michael asked if he could walk her back to her hotel.

"Of course," she said with a smile. "I'd like that."

Michael did not have anything particularly in mind. He had just enjoyed being in the company of a beautiful woman and he was loathe for it to end. When they arrived at her hotel, she asked him if he would like to have another drink—in her room.

Although he considered saying no, he couldn't think of a reason not to go upstairs.

Up in her room, they drank brandy and continued their conversation, talking about the museums and theater in New York. For his part, Michael was having trouble taking his eyes off her lovely figure. When she turned sideways, he traced the outline of her breasts with his eyes. He had a warm feeling regarding the direction the evening was headed.

But then a chilling thought—what if she was sick? What if she had HIV? Although she looked clean, he knew enough to know that looks could be deceiving....

Although concerned, the evening continued. Their conversation turned from the City to more personal matters. He told her about the change in his relationship with his wife.

"I mean, I think it's great that she's so committed to being such a good mother," he said, feeling the need to defend Cindi. "I love her. I do." He lowered his eyes. "I.. I.." he raised his eyes. "You are really very beautiful but I am not interested in going where the evening seems to be headed..."

Elissa smiled a knowing smile. "You are frightened of your wife."

"No, I'm not," Michael said defensively.

"Of course you are. I can hear it in your voice. You are worried about her finding out... or about what she would think..."

"No, that's not it at all," he said.

"No? Then prove it," she said in a voice that was at once both challenging and seductive.

Michael looked at me. "Maybe it was the alcohol. Maybe it was the combination of the warm, island air. The drink. Her beauty. Feeling relaxed for the first time in months... I don't know. But I threw myself on her like an animal. I was going to show her that I didn't have to answer to my wife..."

He was kissing her hair. His hands roamed her body at will. Then Elissa whispered to him not to rush. "We have all the time in the world," she promised.

She went to the bedside table and slid open the drawer. Slowly, she brought out a large vibrator. "Do you know what this is?" she asked teasingly.

"Of course I do," he said, his eyes wide.

"I'll bet your wife hasn't put on a show like this for you in a long time—if ever." With those words, she undressed herself slowly and then, in front of Michael, she began to masturbate. First with her fingertips and then with the vibrator. In only a few moments, she was breathing hard. She sighed loudly and then screamed in three broken screams. "Oh, God..." she whimpered. "Oh, God..."

She was far from finished. She opened her eyes and looked at Michael. "Take off your clothes," she instructed him.

He did as she said.

"Umm," she said, seeing that he had an erection. "Come closer." She reached out and took his erection in her grip, guiding it to her vagina. "Kiss me!" she begged insistently. "Kiss me." A minute later, she took him out of her vagina and moved his penis to her mouth. As she sucked on his penis, she inserted a small dildo into her ass and then inserted the vibrator into her vagina.

In only a few minutes, she was coming again as he ejaculated into her mouth.

"Sure," he told me, "the sex was unbelievable. And there was no money involved. This wasn't a prostitution thing at all... I felt good about that. But the next day I felt guilty as hell. What would I tell my wife? Should I tell my wife? All I could think about in the morning was what I had done and what it might cost me.

"But by early afternoon, I was thinking of Elissa again. I was just so damned attracted to her. I decided I would look for her. Not that that was difficult. She was in the same bar, in the exact same place, as she'd been for the past few evenings."

Michael greeted her warmly.

"It's nice to see you," she said, smiling.

There was a brief moment of awkwardness.

"You were really wonderful yesterday," Michael said.

"You were very good too," she said.

As they sat together, she told him a little about herself. She was a magazine editor, married with two children.

"But... I would have thought... I mean..." Michael stammered. "What kind of relationship do you have with your husband?" he asked. "Are there problems?"

She shook her head. "No, everything is wonderful. We have a very honest and open relationship. I will tell you all about it one day."

Michael was happy not to pursue the subject.

They went to the beach and swam all day. The sun on his back felt so wonderful. When she offered to put suntan lotion on him, she rubbed it in so seductively that he found that he was getting an erection.

When the sun began to go down, they decided to leave the beach.

"Would you like to have dinner together?" Michael asked.

"I'd like that very much."

At dinner, Elissa invited Michael back up to her room. He didn't hesitate, despite the guilt he had felt earlier in the day.

That night, in her room, they engaged in a broader spectrum of sexual activity. Leaning back on her bed, Elissa spread her legs and, as she dragged her finger slowly across the folds of her vagina, she asked him to lick her. He was happy to oblige.

She pressed the back of his head so that his tongue was flush with her clitoris. "Oh, oh, oh," she cried out, having one orgasm after another. When she finally eased the pressure on his head, she smiled at him.

"Now, let me do something I'll bet you've never done before."

"What's that?" he asked.

"Just lay back and enjoy it."

As he lay on his back, Elissa straddled his thighs and dipped her fingertips into some oil she kept by the bed. Then she massaged the oil onto his penis and balls. When he was so greased up that his penis glistened, she lifted herself up and, reaching back and taking his penis, eased herself down while guiding him into her ass.

He groaned with pleasure as he felt the exquisite tightness.

She maintained control of the pace. Soon, they were both ready to explode.

They spent the remaining days of his vacation/business trip enjoying each other. But finally, the day came for his departure.

"I.. I don't know what to say," he told her honestly. "These have been some of the most wonderful days I can remember..."

She smiled and kissed him. "Don't say anything," she said. "Take this." she handed him a piece of paper on which she had written her telephone number. "When I get home, I'd like to invite you to come out to Short Hills and meet my husband..."

He looked at her like she was out of her mind. What did she expect, that he would reciprocate and invite her to meet his wife? No way! She had to be joking.

When he returned to New York, he discovered that nothing had changed in his relationship with his wife. His absence had not made her any more anxious to rekindle the sexual fires they had once enjoyed. Still, his sexual escapade with Elissa had given him a great deal of satisfaction and he wasn't overly anxious to have sex. In addition, work hit him like a ton of bricks and he was once again working long hours, seven days a week.

No more swims in the morning or evenings in the bar with Elissa...

"But then," he told me, "three weeks later, I couldn't stand it anymore. I had kept the piece of paper from Elissa in my office—I wouldn't have dared to keep it at home. What if Cindi would have found it?

"Anyway, I phoned Elissa. She sounded glad to hear from me. She invited me to her house for dinner. She said that her husband wanted to meet me.

"There it was again—her husband. It just didn't make sense. I didn't know what to make of it. I dismissed it to her being a joker. You know, having that as a line when we met and then following it through. I don't know..."

A few days later, having made his excuses to Cindi, Michael headed to Short Hills and Elissa's house. He arrived promptly at eight o'clock, as she had requested. He had flowers and champagne. He rang the door bell. A moment later, the door opened and he found himself looking at a man, fairly nice looking, about fifty years old.

"I'm.. I'm sorry," he stammered. "I.. I must have the wrong address."

The man shook his head and smiled with a knowing, sarcastic smile. "No, no. You're in the right place. Come on in. Elissa will be back in a few minutes. She just had to run to the store." When Michael hesitated, the man urged him to come in. "Don't be embarrassed. Really."

Michael didn't know what to think. He couldn't imagine that this guy was really Elissa's husband. What kind of man let his wife behave like she had behaved? Even if this was the nineties, there were some things that just weren't right...

"Have a seat," the man said, showing Michael into a comfortable den.

"Thanks," Michael said.

Michael didn't know what to say. They were both quiet for the several minutes.

"How about something to drink?" the man suggested.

"That would be great," Michael agreed.

It was a few more minutes before Elissa came in. When she saw Michael, she smiled. "I see you've met," she said.

Michael smiled uncomfortably. The man got up to go to the kitchen and to get another champagne glass for Elissa. When he was gone, Elissa looked at Michael.

"Let me tell you what's happening," she said, her voice earnest and direct. "Two years ago, my husband was in a terrible car accident. For a short time, the doctors weren't sure if he would survive. Thankfully, he made it. But there were some lasting injuries. One of them is that he was rendered impotent." She paused. She smiled tightly. "We used to love each other and still do love each other very much. We're very close. Maybe in some ways closer than we used to be." She sighed. "We always enjoyed such wonderful sex. I..as you probably have come to realize, I very much enjoy sex.

"There is just no way that I could remain celibate for the rest of my life. So, in order to avoid divorcing, we decided that it was better for me to have a lover to take care of my sexual needs. That," she added, glancing down at her hands, "was the agreement.

"So I took a lover. Before you, there was one man. I ended our relationship a month ago. I was looking for someone else when I met you. I thought you would be a very good person..."

Michael listened but only half understood. The combination of the champagne, being close to Elissa again and the strangeness of the circumstances disoriented him and made it difficult for him to grasp what she was saying. He thought that maybe she was still joking.

"Great, great," he said. "You husband is wonderful."

The whole thing was like a strange dream to him. He continued to drink until the bottle of champagne was finished.

"Come," Elissa said, standing up and extending her hand to him. "Let's go enjoy each other."

Before leading him to her bedroom, Elissa went to the kitchen where she took some ice cream from the freezer. Then she led the way into the bedroom. She quickly undressed and put dollops of ice cream on different parts of her body. On her breasts, between her breasts, on her navel, in her pubic hair and inside her vagina.

"Come along, lover," she sighed. "Enjoy your dessert."

Michael, horny from the champagne and now from seeing Elissa writhing on the bed. He quickly stripped off her clothes and jumped onto the bed. He ate the ice cream, licking it off her breasts and belly and then nestling himself between her legs where the touch of his tongue drove her wild.

"Oh, oh, oh.."

She screamed and sighed. Soon, she was whimpering with pleasure. She flipped over onto her belly. Michael reached his hands under her hips and lifted her ass into the air. Using some ice cream as a lubricant, he thrust his erection into her ass, repeating the success he'd enjoyed in Puerto Rico.

Soon, she was screaming and begging him to thrust harder and harder. In a few moments, they both came together.

Michael slid off her and laid on his back, breathing deeply. Elissa was only just getting warmed up. While Michael regained his strength, she took her vibrator. She rubbed it over her nipples and then over her clitoris.

"Do me with it," she begged Michael. "Please. Do me."

He took the vibrator and inserted it into her vagina. Soon, he was fucking her with the vibrator as she pinched her nipples. After coming several times, she lay back on the bed and caught her breath.

She got up and brought them some coffee. As they were in bed, drinking the coffee, she asked him if he wanted to see a movie.

He shrugged, not knowing what to think. "Sure," he said.

The man who had greeted him at the door came in the bedroom. Michael quickly covered himself up. A few minutes later, he realized just how stupid his modesty was. The man slipped a VCR into the player. In a moment, Michael realized the movie that he was watching was a movie of him and Elissa.

"What the fuck?" he cried out. "What is this?" he demanded. "You're crazy, you know that?" he said to Elissa. "This was private, not a show!"

Elissa looked shocked. "I've told you the truth. This man is my husband..."

Michael was mad as hell. He got dressed and stormed out of the house. Although he'd had much too much to drink, he somehow made it back to New York. He wanted nothing so much as to fall asleep and pretend the evening never happened. But he couldn't fall asleep. He took some pills to help him relax and, as a reward for the pills and the drinking and the carousing, he woke up the following morning with a splitting headache.

As mad as he was, time softened his anger. Nothing changed in his relationship with his wife. Two weeks later, he phone Elissa. She couldn't have been more apologetic. She was practically in tears.

Michael went to see her again. When they met face to face, she broke down in tears and begged him to forgive her. "This isn't the way I wanted my life to be," she told him.

He forgave her. He understood finally that she was telling the truth and that the man was her husband. He couldn't help but think that life must be a living hell for him.

Michael continued to see Elissa every week for over six

months—on the condition that they make no more tapes. However, he arrived at my office with a yellow discharge from his penis and experiencing pain when he urinated.

"What's the matter with me, doc?" he asked urgently. "What's going on? Can you help me?"

After a thorough examination and lab work, the diagnosis was nongonoccal tetritus. I was able to treat Michael successfully. However, about three weeks after I saw him last, I received a frantic phone call from him.

"I have to see you as soon as possible," he said over the phone.

"What's the matter?" I asked him.

"I'll explain when I see you."

I had my receptionist schedule the earliest possible appointment for him the following day. When he came in, I could see he was nervous and upset.

"About two weeks after I finished the treatment," he said, "I had this sharp pain in my right hand and left foot," he said, extending his hand as if in proof. "And then this..."

He stuck out his tongue, displaying that there was erosion of the tongue. As I looked more closely at him, I could see that his eyes were red as well—a symptom that I had attributed to his being tired when he first came in.

I brought him into the examination room. Upon close examination, I discovered a number of shallow erosions on his penis. Inspection of his tongue showed red-gray spotting. When I examined his hand and foot, he jerked them back in pain.

He was suffering from severe inflammation in both—arthritis. The redness in his eyes was the result of conjunctivitis. Subsequent blood work showed that he was suffering from mild anemia and that his white blood count was elevated.

Based on all this evidence, I diagnosed acute Reiter's syndrome, a condition in which there is a combination of arthritis and urethritis. Often, there is accompanying conjunctivitis. It usually develops following nonspecific urethritis.

I immediately began to treat him. I also suggested that he get in touch with Elissa.

Hearing the news, Elissa agreed to come in to be examined. Upon my examination and lab work, I diagnosed active arthritis in her as well. She also had a bacterial urinary infection.

Like with Michael, I was able to successfully treat her. She remained under my care and supervision until all her symptoms disappeared.

Michael and Elissa's situation is a powerful one. Unique perhaps, in that they were both "in the same place", for similar reasons but with different causes. Both sought out (Elissa more actively than Michael, perhaps) sexual encounters outside of their marriage because their marriages were not fulfilling their sexual needs. In Elissa's case, this was because her husband, a man she loved very deeply, was no longer able to perform sexually as the result of injuries sustained in a car accident.

Michael's wife, whom he loved both as his wife and as the mother of his children, also failed to engage in satisfactory sexual relations with her husband. If she had, it is unlikely that he would have sought sexual gratification elsewhere. Her reasons might have been hormonal, following the birth of their second child. They might have been psychological. However, the end result was that Michael felt compelled to seek sexual gratification in another person's arms.

This is very often the case—especially in marriages where the partners are still physically attractive, as Michael viewed

Cindi. She was fit. Healthy. Pretty. She simply "lost interest". As a result, Michael sought "interest" someplace else.

Elissa found herself in a position that she never wanted nor invited. Only an understanding husband allowed her to find gratification that he *could* not provide. Cindi *would* not engage in sexual encounters with her husband, essentially forcing him to seek comfort elsewhere.

I don't present these two situations in order to offer a "moral comparison". Rather, to demonstrate the importance of satisfactory sexual relations within marriage (or any other monogamous relationship.) The safest sex is, of course, no sex at all. However, few individuals would opt for that degree of safety. Instead, most people would be happy to enjoy a satisfactory sexual experience with their spouse.

It seems that, when *that* falls short—for whatever reasons—people seek other sexual gratification. And it is here, in a more promiscuous setting, that it is more difficult to engage in "safe sex".

23

WHEN SEX SHOULDN'T HAPPEN—AND THE CONSEQUENCES

We have sexual relations for many, many reasons. These relations take on many different forms—they might be monogamous, homosexual, heterosexual, fleeting, long-lasting, involve multiple partners, involve "kinky" sex, or be just straight, missionary intercourse. I have stated repeatedly in this book that a healthy sexual appetite is the result of being a healthy human being. I have also pointed out that sex, while sometimes very simple and straightforward, calls into play a complex interplay of emotion, hormones, history and experience. Most of these things are to the good. Sometimes, they are damaging and destructive.

In short, not all sex is good. Not all sex is appropriate. Not all sex should happen. And in these observations, I am not referring to sex being "safe" or not.

When Olney came to my office, I knew immediately that there was a great deal going on beyond whatever physical symptoms she would present to me. She was seated but clearly agitated. Her eyes moved around the room quickly. When they settled on me, her expression hovered between need and distrust.

"How can I help you?" I asked simply.

She glanced down at the floor and then up at me. It seemed that my question, viewed by so many as an invitation to describe symptoms, opened a floodgate of memories and feelings for her.

"I'm a slut," she said boldly. She watched me closely, measuring my reaction.

"Why would you say that?" I asked her after a moment.

"Because I'll fuck anything," she replied. Then her expression showed the struggle she was fighting between anger and hurt. "My father raped me—pure and simple," she said, her anger winning out. "I was fourteen."

I waited. In the next couple of seconds, I remember being exquisitely conscious of the near-silence in the room. Only Olney's ragged breathing interrupted that silence. "One night... he came home drunk..." She raised her eyes and looked at me. "We weren't what you'd call a model family," she noted with a great deal of irony. "We had lots of problems. My mother and father didn't get along at all. They stayed together. That's the most you could say for them. They went through the motions. But they didn't love each other. They hardly liked each other.

"That was obvious to me... even when I was really young. They didn't even sleep together. I mean, I can't be sure. I didn't sleep in the same room with them. But if I had to bet... " She shrugged. "Maybe my father drank to numb himself. I don't know. How the hell would I know?

"I mean, if you knew his family you'd understand why he

was always pissed off. They were always arguing, always putting each other down. They never said a nice thing to one another. No praise. Nothing.

"My father just didn't like my mother. Me, I was the one who was on the receiving end of his anger." Her eyes filled up. "I guess he wanted a perfect daughter, you know. Maybe he figured that would shut his family up. But I wasn't perfect. No one is.

"If ... whenever I fucked up... watch out! I'd catch it. Of course, when I did things right, nothing. When I got good grades, he didn't say a word. And then, listen to this, this is really the kicker, he would give me stuff for doing *nothing*. You know, just out of nowhere. You figure that out.

"I've been in therapy for years now and I still can't figure out his brilliant system of disincentive.

"Not that I didn't always try to be his model daughter. I think I fell in love with sports for him..."

Olney, at thirty-six, was an attractive woman who wrote for a national sports magazine.

She waved her hand gently in front of her. "I won't bother going into the gory details of the rape or the years of incest... maybe just a couple." She looked at me and then quickly looked away. "He was really drunk. Staggering almost. Making more noise when he tried not to. Anyway, I was in bed and he came into my bedroom and just jumped on me.

"Shit, I was just a girl. He was this man. I remember thinking, Where's my mother? But I didn't have much time to think about anything other than what he was doing to me. He was hurting me. And then he grabbed my pajama top. I was old enough to know what he was getting at when he tore my pajamas off me and pressed his hand over my mouth.

"I was scared. I was embarrassed. I mean, my father was in my bed and I wasn't wearing any clothes. I didn't even have tits yet... it was horrible. And I could hardly breath.

"He pushed my legs apart... I remember hitting him, scratching him, trying to bite his hand, kicking him... but nothing mattered. He was going to do what he was going to do. He stuck it in me and the pain paralyzed me.

"He fucked me real hard and real fast..." she shook her head. "After that, it was a regular thing. He would come into my bedroom..." her voice was barely louder than a whisper. "Did I say I was fourteen? I couldn't have been that old. I bet I wasn't even twelve yet. Probably barely eleven." Olney looked up at me. "Not a very pleasant way to lose your virginity, I'll tell you that." She snorted bitterly. "I remember being in the locker room at school and overhearing these girls talking about their dates and how far they should go. How they'd get all weird if a guy tried to touch their breasts and how they'd *never* let a guy touch them *down there.*

"And the thought of going all the way..." Olney leaned back and looked up at the ceiling. She let a long breath out through her pursed lips. "Man, if only I could have had the worries that they had. For them, losing their virginity was a whole ritual they were a part of—even if they tried to play innocent. They were mostly cock teases but you can't imagine how I wished I could have been just like them.

"When I got to college, I had lots and lots of boyfriends. Nearly all of them were angry young men who drank too much." She laughed bitterly and smeared some tears with the heel of her hand. Her cheek glistened with the moisture. "Sigmund Freud, are you listening? Jesus, I was a regular whore in college.

"Some kids spent their free time in the library. I spent mine in one bed or another. I sucked and fucked my way through those years. I wish they gave credit for blowjobs. I would have graduated with high honors.

"I had quite the reputation, as you can imagine," she added with ironic understatement. "And you know what? All the girls who I knew who were so scared of having a reputation? Well, I wasn't one of them. I *loved* being known as the campus slut. I loved taking on all comers. I didn't care. Big cock. Small cock. Experienced. Inexperienced. Handsome. Ugly. Fat. Athletic... They were all just bodies attached to dicks.

"Of course, even I couldn't stomach myself *all* the time. There were plenty of times I was disgusted with myself and my life. God, how I hated myself then." She turned away and looked toward the window in my office. "If I could have changed my life..." She turned back and looked at me. "I would have done anything to make everything different," she said urgently. "But I couldn't," she added, sounding defeated.

"There was one guy during my junior year... he was a lovely guy. Sweet. Caring. He was a philosophy major. I don't know how I ended up with him. I didn't meet him the way I met most guys—at a bar or a fraternity party. I think he spoke to me during a class we both had.

"It was so.. so nice. So normal. I was with him for about six months. We held hands. We didn't fuck so much as make love. He was great. Gentle. Caring. He did things *for me.*

"I wanted to marry him. You know, get married and put an end to the whole business of my life." She shrugged. "Sort of retire to a quiet domesticity." She clasped her hands and leaned forward. "We used to visit jewelry stores and shop for rings. I mean, he loved me. At least, he told me he did.

"We bought rings too. We bought wedding rings," she went on, emphasizing the kind of ring as if to remind herself that it had actually happened. "But I backed out at the last minute. I just couldn't give up my life of addiction," she added smugly. Then her voice changed. "I didn't deserve him," she said flatly. "He was too good. Too decent. I was... I was who I was."

Olney explained how, after that, she didn't have much stomach for college. "Never did get my degree," she observed. However, she had created a network of sorts. Through the athletes she'd had sex with in college, she came to meet—and party with—professional athletes.

"Oh, I fucked them all. You name them, I fucked them. Baseball. Football. Basketball. I was a regular groupie.

"I got my job writing thanks to one of those guys." She looked at my slyly. "Do you want to know who it was?"

I shook my head. "No. No, thank you." I leaned forward a little and looked Olney directly in the eye. "Tell me, why have you come to visit me?"

She drew a deep breath. She thought for a moment, as if deciding where to start this most recent part of her story. If nothing else, her story made a compelling case for believing who we are is the sum total of our experiences, of who we've been.

"I was doing this guy from the office," she began slowly. "Nothing heavy. He's a golf writer, for god's sake. I mean, he wears those pastel colors and shit. But he appeals to me. When I first got him in bed, he was a real dud. Straight in and out kind of guy.

"I had to teach him everything. Like, when I first brought up the idea of anal he completely freaked out. He's like most guys though... it doesn't take much convincing to get them in that back door. I like that a lot. I really do. Some girls say they like it but don't. I *really* do.

"Anyway, this guy hadn't had a lot of experience with oral either. I loved licking his balls while he had his tongue up me.

"Once he started getting the hang of it, he was a real bull. We'd do it on the living room floor. I still have carpet burns on my butt." She chuckled. "Then there's this girl I met from college." She stopped and looked at me. "I mean, *she's* a college student. I never went back to college. As I told you, my major was sex, my minor was alcohol.

"Anyway, Liz is this real cute thing... I spotted her at the YMCA after an aerobics class. She was taking a shower right next to me and it was all I could do to keep myself from reaching out and touching her. What a gorgeous body! The way the soap suds were dripping off her...ummm." She closed her eyes and seemed to relish in the memory. "Did I tell you that I went both ways?" she asked, opening her eyes again.

Olney described her relationship with Liz in complete graphic detail. "I don't know, maybe I like women because they've never been mean to me," she observed. "Maybe I just like the softness of a woman's touch... or her skin next to mine.

"The first time I licked another woman... it was the most wonderful thing. And feeling a woman's fingers on my clit... so knowing and fluttery. Ooh. Liz was amazing. We used to do each other up the butt with our vibrators when we were doing a sixty-nine. You can't imagine how good that felt..."

"Do you still speak with your parents?" I asked.

She stopped. "I talk to my mother a couple of times a week. We're on pretty good terms. We probably get along better now than we ever did. Of course, both me and my father made her promise never to say anything about the rape and stuff. I think that really bothers her, how all that happened and she didn't do anything to stop it. But what could she do? My father was a fucking angry drunk..."

Olney told me about the numerous abortions she'd had over the years. "Could you imagine me as a mother?" she asked, laughing in a self-depreciating manner.

"You know, sometimes I think my best sex partner is myself. One my favorite things to do is to gather some of my vibrators and dildos and to get in front of a mirror and do myself... Jerkoff Theater," she concluded with a chuckle. Then her voice darkened. "I know that two of my lovers have died from AIDS," she said. She shook her head. "They ended up as drug users as well."

She drew a deep breath. "Anyway, listen to me talking so much. I came here because I have this itching when I pee and the stuff coming out of my vagina..." she made a face. "It makes some stink. And I just feel lousy, like I've got the flu or something." She started slipping her shoe off. "I've got this rash that spreads all over my body but it's real bad on the soles of my feet."

I listened as Olney explained her symptoms and then we went into the examination room. Although there was some sign of rash and some discharge, she was virtually symptom free.

"You mean, there's nothing wrong with me?" she asked, grinning.

"Nothing I can find right now," I told her. I did some lab tests. A culture and some blood work. An HIV test. "We should know more when the tests come back from the lab."

Three days later, when I received the lab report for Olney, we did know more, much more. Olney had tested positive for HIV.

When I told her, her shoulders sagged. "I got the AIDS?"

"At this point, you have the virus that causes AIDS, yes," I said.

She started to cry softly. I went over and put my hand on her shoulder.

"It's not fair," she said. "It's just not fair."

Some might argue that she, of all people, could not make that argument. That she had spent her entire adult life engaging in unsafe, promiscuous sex. Some might argue that for her AIDS was an expected outcome.

It is true Olney was an adult. She was able to make choices. However, no one should ever forget that on a particular night during her *childhood* her father, drunk and himself suffering from years of unhappy living, came into her bedroom and raped her. And that that rape was followed by years of incestuous sexual activity.

Olney was a victim of sex that should never happen. And anyone who judges her behavior as an adult without acknowledging that truth, without taking it into account, is worse than a fool.

I have met too many people who have expressed, in dangerous sexual practices, a lack of self-esteem which resulted from too many years of being put down, abused, or mocked.

They inevitably pay for their behavior in one way or another but it is important to understand that their behavior is itself a payment of sorts. As Olney cried that day, saying over and over, "It isn't fair" she was one hundred percent correct. It was unfair that a satisfying, self-respected life should have always remained just beyond her grasp.

And always would.

One year from when she first came to my office, Olney died. Another victim of AIDS.

Conclusion

When I return to my home at the end of the day, driving along the street and past the houses with their fine lawns and blossoming flowers, the houses that "protect" their inhabitants from the horrible diseases that I treat every day, the first thing I do is wash my hands. Not because they are dirty but because the ritual of hand washing, a ritual that I engage in so many times during the day, calms me, helps me to separate my home life from my life with my patients.

But I am not deluded, as so many of my neighbors are. Having a clean bathroom in a nice house to wash my hands affords me no protection from the diseases that I see and treat every day. I am as vulnerable as anyone else.

Knowledge. Safe-sex practices. These are the only protections we have.

There is no "wrong" sex. Just as there is no "right" sex. There is sex. People engage in sex for all sorts of reasons. Some good. Some bad. My hope and goal is that, regardless of the particular experience, the participants live long and healthy so that they may learn from it. Just as I would hope we all learn from our experiences.

The first lesson is that it can happen to anyone. You and me. It is a lesson none of us can afford to forget.